Stanley McDowell

101 Delicious E-Liquid Recipes
How to Save Money by Making Your Own DIY Vape E-Juice in 4 Easy Steps

Table of Contents

INTRODUCTION

First of all, I would like to thank you for downloading the book, "101 Delicious E-Liquid Recipes: How to Save Money by Making Your Own DIY Vape E-Juice in 4 Easy Steps."

Mixing your own e-liquid can be an interesting, weird, frustrating, fun journey, depending on how much knowledge and patience you have. If it's your first time mixing, you probably have loads of questions. To put your mind at ease, we've made a tutorial with 4 easy steps to create your own e-liquid.

It's a very simple process. You can customize e-juice to your own taste and control how much nicotine you get. We're going to demonstrate how to make delicious cookie flavour – Hoochie Cookies. This is one of our all-day vape recipes!

Flavor Supplier Abbreviations:

CAP – Capella

FA – Flavour Art

TPA/TFA – The Perfumer's Apprentice/The Flavor Apprentice

FW – Flavor West

INA/INW – Inawera

Misc. DIY Abbreviations:

AP – Acetyl Pyrazine

EM – Ethyl Maltol

PG – Propylene Glycol

VG – Vegetable Glycerin

HOW TO MAKE VAPE JUICE IN 4 EASY STEPS

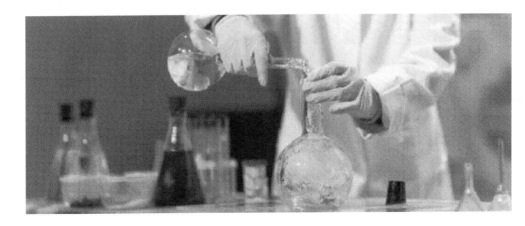

STEP 1. PREPARE FLAVORS

The first step is to find a recipe, and then buy the relevant concentrates. Don't forget to shake them well before mixing! For this example, we'll use the recipe for <u>Hoochie Cookies</u>, a delicious cookie flavour created by our team:

CAP Sugar Cookie 6%

FW Butter Pecan 4%

FW White Chocolate 3%

TPA Bavarian Cream 2%

FA Cinnamon Ceylon 0,5%

FA Marshmallow 1%

CAP Super Sweet 0,75%

TPA Acetyl Pyrazine 5 PG 1%

Well, you can do no wrong with bavarian cream and white chocolate combined with sugar cookie and butter pecan. At least not in our Recipe Book.

STEP 2. PREPARE BASE

The second step is to find the ideal ratio between VG and PG, and buy the base. We recommend you use 30/70 PG/VG for all our recipes. Let's look at the picture.

PG to VG Ratios in E-Liquid

PG%	VG%	Vapour Production	Throat Hit
100%	0%	Very little vapour production	Very strong throat hit, maximum level
80%	20%	Very little vapour production	Strong throat hit
70%	30%	Slightly more obvious vapour	Slightly less than strong throat hit
60%	40%	Obvious vapour	Throat hit is no longer overwhelming
50%	50%	Moderate vapour	Moderate throat hit
40%	60%	Larger vapour clouds	Smoother throat hit
30%	70%	Good vapour production	Minimal throat hit
20%	80%	Excellent vapour production	Barely noticeable throat hit
0%	100%	Huge plumes of vapour, much sweeter taste	No throat hit whatsoever

Next, choose your nicotine level. Here, we'll make a 30 mL bottle of Hoochie Cookies, with 3 mg nicotine and PG/VG at a 30/70 ratio.

The strength of the nicotine we're using is 3mg/mL, which means for every milliliter of liquid there are 3 mg of nicotine. Now we need to mix the flavors with the base.

STEP 3. MIX THE BLEND

1. Shake flavors well before using.

2. When you've got everything ready, mix flavors from the picture in a bottle and add 24,53 mL of base (PG+VG+Nicotine).

3. Then shake your bottle, and I mean shake it VERY well. The final weight should match that shown on the eLR table.

4. Place your bottle of e-liquid in a dark place for 21 days. That's all!

Ingredient	ml	Grams	%
■ Nicotine juice 100 mg (30/70 PG/VG)	0.90	**1.07**	3.00
■ PG dilutant	3.26	**3.38**	10.87
■ VG dilutant	20.37	**25.69**	67.90
Total base	*24.53*	*30.14*	*81.77*
Acetyl Pyrazine 5% (TPA)	0.30	**0.30**	1.00
⚠ Bavarian Cream (TPA)	0.60	**0.60**	2.00
Butter Pecan (FW)	1.20	**1.20**	4.00
Cinnamon Ceylon (FA)	0.15	**0.15**	0.50
Marshmallow (FA)	0.30	**0.30**	1.00
⚠ Sugar Cookie (CAP)	1.80	**1.80**	6.00
Super Sweet (CAP)	0.23	**0.23**	0.75
White Chocolate (FW)	0.90	**0.90**	3.00
Totals	*30.01*	**35.62**	*100*

Suggested steep time: 21 days

Strength: 3 mg
PG/VG-ratio: 30/70
Flavor total: 5.48 ml / 5.48g (18.25%)

STEP 4. HOW TO STEEP YOUR E-LIQUID

While most liquid manufacturers steep their liquid in advance, many e-liquids will reach you when they are still very freshly made. Steeping allows the ingredients of the e-juice to more thoroughly mix and can give it a more uniform complex and mellow taste.

To steep your e-liquid, all you need to do is leave it in a cool dark place and shake it once every couple of days. You can do this for a few days or up to a month, depending on how much change to the flavour you want to occur. If you want to expedite the steeping process, you can expose your e-liquid to heat. Exposing it to heat energizes its molecules, causing them to move faster, mixing the e-liquid more quickly.

The most common way to expose bottles of e-juice to heat is to soak them in warm water. Place the bottles in water that is 85 to 105 degrees Fahrenheit, and let them soak until the water is at room temperature. It's recommended that you do this with glass bottles, as glass conducts heat more effectively and is more resistance to breaking down over time. In addition to steeping, it's also effective to let your juice breathe.

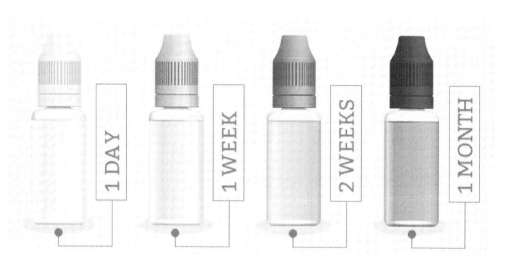

Letting e-liquid breathe is the process of leaving the lid or dripper off of a bottle to intentionally expose it to air. This causes the liquid to oxidize, which can remove the harsh perfume-like taste of freshly mixed e-juice, but it can also cause the nicotine to darken in color and begin breaking down. So it's recommended that you don't leave an e-liquid to breathe for more than a few hours.

While the results will vary, steeping is an effective way to change the flavor of e-juice and a good way to experience new flavour.

Now, let's mix some e-liquid!

CHAPTER 1: OUR TOP 8 PREMIUM E-LIQUID RECIPES

CREAM BASE

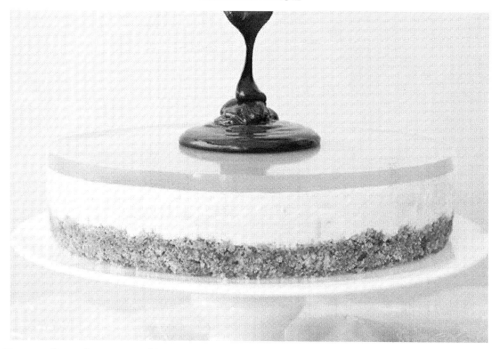

We use base in many e-liquids here.

You can make a large batch of this to save time on mixing later.

FA Catalan Cream 3%

FA Cream Fresh 1%

FA Vienna Cream 2%

FA Custard 2%

FA Marshmallow 1%

Suggested steep time – 21 days. This base is unlike anything you've vaped before. Let's make some fun!

HOOCHIE COOKIE MAN

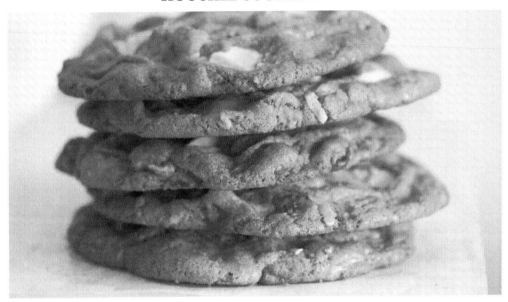

1. Grab your nic base. We recommend you use 70/30 VG/PG.

2. Add these flavours, and shake them well before mixing:

CAP Sugar Cookie 6%

FW Butter Pecan 4%

FW White Chocolate 3%

TPA Bavarian Cream 2%

FA Cinnamon Ceylon 0,5%

FA Marshmallow 1%

CAP Super Sweet 0,75%

TPA Acetyl Pyrazine 5 PG 1%

3. Shake well and place your bottle of e-liquid in a dark place for 21 days. Enjoy vaping your new e-juice!

CHOCOLATE COOKIE ICE CREAM SANDWICH

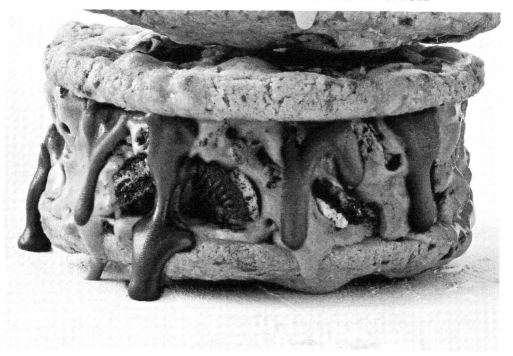

1. Grab your nic base. We recommend you use 70/30 VG/PG.

2. Add these flavours, and shake them well before mixing:

CAP Sugar Cookie 3%

FW Graham Cracker 1%

FW Cookies and Cream 7%

FA Custard 2%

FA Marshmallow 1%

TPA Acetyl Pyrazine 5 PG 1%

TPA Koolada 0,5%

3. Shake well and place your bottle of e-liquid in a dark place for 21 days. Enjoy vaping your new e-juice!

BOURBON-BUTTER PECAN ICE CREAM

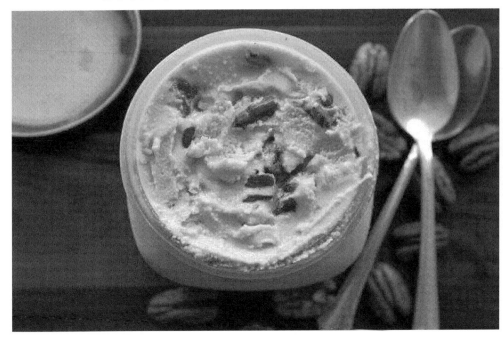

1. Grab your nic base. We recommend you use 70/30 VG/PG.

2. Add these flavours, and shake them well before mixing:

FW Butter Pecan 4%

TPA Kentucky Bourbon 2%

FA Catalan Cream 3%

FA Cream Fresh 1%

FA Vienna Cream 2%

FA Custard 2%

FA Marshmallow 1%

CAP Super Sweet 0,75%

3. Shake well and place your bottle of e-liquid in a dark place for 21-28 days. Enjoy vaping your new e-juice!

MOCHA BROWNIE ICE CREAM CAKE

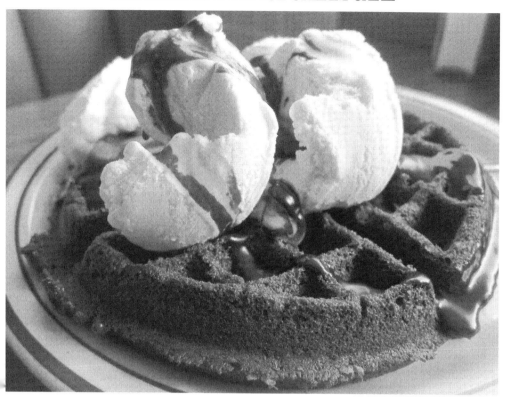

1. Grab your nic base. We recommend you use 70/30 VG/PG.

2. Add these flavours, and shake them well before mixing:

FW Yellow Cake 2%

CAP Cake Batter 1%

CAP Chocolate Fudge Brownie 4%

FA Cream Fresh 1%

FA Vienna Cream 2%

FA Custard 2%

FA Marshmallow 1%

CAP Super Sweet 0,75%

TPA Acetyl Pyrazine 5 PG 1%

3. Shake well and place your bottle of e-liquid in a dark place for 28 days. Enjoy vaping your new e-juice!

CHOCOLATE PANCAKE WITH RASPBERRIES AND FRESH CREAM

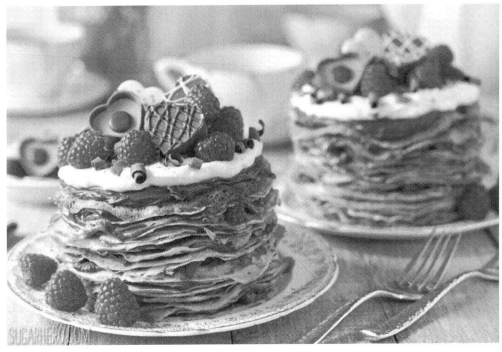

1. Grab your nic base. We recommend you use 70/30 VG/PG.

2. Add these flavours, and shake them well before mixing:

TPA Pancakes 2%

TPA Butter 0.2%

CAP Raspberry v2 1.75%

FA Fresh Cream 1.5%

FA Marshmallow 1%

FA Tiramisu 0.5%

FA Torrone 0,5%

FW White Chocolate 2%

TPA Acetyl Pyrazine 5 PG 0,5%

3. Shake well and place your bottle of e-liquid in a dark place for 21-28 days. Enjoy vaping your new e-juice!

CINNAMON ROLL WAFFLE ICE CREAM SANDWICHES

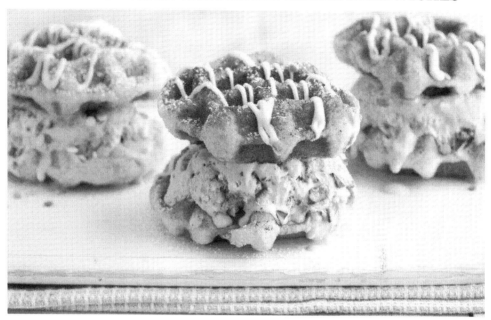

1. Grab your nic base. We recommend you use 70/30 VG/PG.

2. Add these flavours, and shake them well before mixing:

TPA Waffle (Belgian) 5%

FA Cinnamon Ceylon 0,25%

FA Cream Fresh 1%

FA Vienna Cream 2%

FA Custard 2%

FA Marshmallow 1%

FA Butterscotch 0,5%

TPA Malted Milk 0,5%

TPA Acetyl Pyrazine 5 PG 1%

CAP Super Sweet 0,75%

3. Shake well and place your bottle of e-liquid in a dark place for 21 days. Enjoy vaping your new e-juice!

BANANA-RUM ICE CREAM

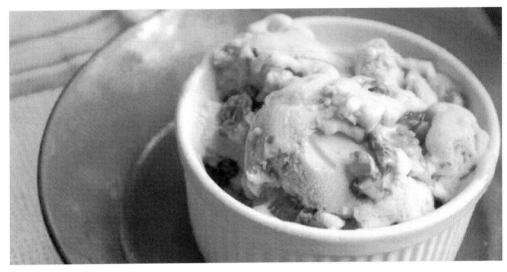

1. Grab your nic base. We recommend you use 70/30 VG/PG.

2. Add these flavours, and shake them well before mixing:

TPA Banana Cream 5%

FA Custard 3%

FA Jamaican Rum 2% or 3%, depending on your taste.

TPA Malted Milk 0,5%

FA Butterscotch 0,5%

FA Marshmallow 1%

CAP French Vanilla 1%

FA Maple Syrup 0,25%

CAP Super Sweet 0,75%

TPA Koolada 0,5%

3. Shake well and place your bottle of e-liquid in a dark place for 14-21 days. Enjoy vaping your new e-juice!

BELGIAN WAFFLE WITH BANANA ICE CREAM AND MAPLE SYRUP

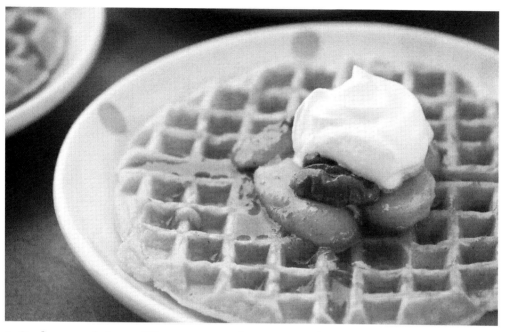

1. Grab your nic base. We recommend you use 70/30 VG/PG.

2. Add these flavours, and shake them well before mixing:

TPA Waffle (Belgian) 6%

TPA Banana Cream 4%

FA Vienna Cream 2%

FA Fresh Cream 1%

FA Jamaican Rum 2%

FA Marshmallow 1%

FA Maple Syrup 0,25%

TPA Acetyl Pyrazine 5 PG 1%

3. Shake well and place your bottle of e-liquid in a dark place for 21-28 days. Enjoy vaping your new e-juice!

CHAPTER 2: DESSERT RECIPES

TIRAMISU ICE CREAM SANDWICH

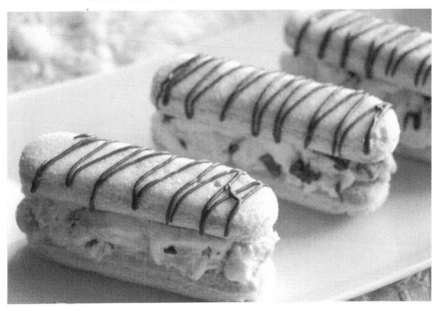

1. Grab your nic base. We recommend you use 70/30 VG/PG.

2. Add these flavours, and shake them well before mixing:

FA Cookie 1%

TPA Graham Cracker 2%

FA Catalan Cream 3%

FA Cream Fresh 1%

FA Vienna Cream 2%

FA Custard 2%

FA Tiramisu 1%

FA Marshmallow 1%

CAP Super Sweet 0,75%

TPA Acetyl Pyrazine 5 PG 1%

3. Shake well and place your bottle of e-liquid in a dark place for 21 days. Enjoy vaping your new e-juice!

PARIS BREST WITH COFFEE CREAM

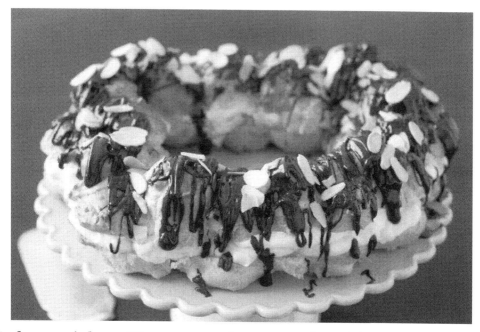

1. Grab your nic base. We recommend you use 70/30 VG/PG.

2. Add these flavours, and shake them well before mixing:

CAP Churro 3%

FA Zeppola 2%

CAP Cake Batter 1%

FA Custard 1%

CAP Golden Butter 0,5%

FA Irish Cream 1,5%

TPA Bavarian Cream 2%

FA Marshmallow 1%

CAP Super Sweet 0,75%

TPA Acetyl Pyrazine 5 PG 1%

3. Shake well and place your bottle of e-liquid in a dark place for 28 days. Enjoy vaping your new e-juice!

PARIS BREST WITH STRAWBERRY

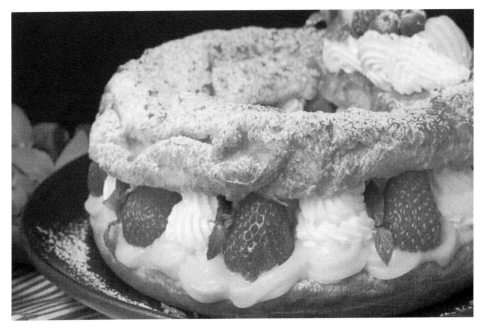

1. Grab your nic base. We recommend you use 70/30 VG/PG.

2. Add these flavours, and shake them well before mixing:

FA wOw 3,5%

FA Zeppola 2,5% or 3%. Depending on your taste.

CAP Sweet Strawberry 3%

TPA Strawberry Ripe 2%

FA Custard 1%

TPA Bavarian Cream 2%

FA Torrone 0,75%

FA Meringue 2%

FA Marshmallow 1%

CAP Super Sweet 0,75%

TPA Acetyl Pyrazine 5 PG 1%

3. Shake well and place your bottle of e-liquid in a dark place for 28 days. Enjoy vaping your new e-juice!

CHOCOLATE CROISSANT

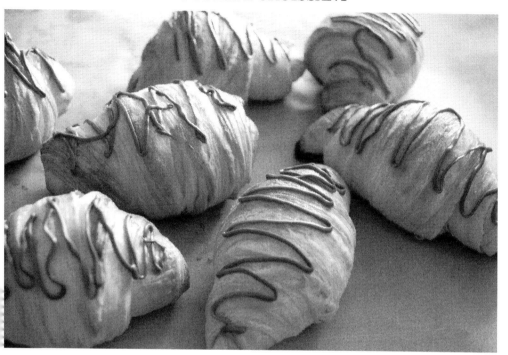

1. Grab your nic base. We recommend you use 70/30 VG/PG.

2. Add these flavours, and shake them well before mixing:

CAP Churro 2%

FA Zeppola 3%

TPA Double Chocolate Clear 2%

TPA Vanilla Swirl 1,5%

FA Torrone 0,75%

FA Meringue 2%

FA Marshmallow 1%

CAP Super Sweet 0,75%

TPA Acetyl Pyrazine 5 PG 1%

3. Shake well and place your bottle of e-liquid in a dark place for 21 days. Enjoy vaping your new e-juice!

CROISSANT WITH RASPBERRY JAM

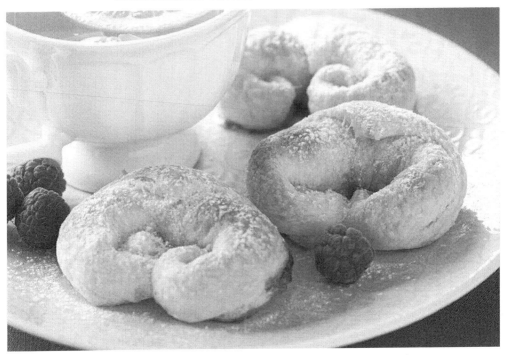

1. Grab your nic base. We recommend you use 70/30 VG/PG.

2. Add these flavours, and shake them well before mixing:

FA Zeppola 3%

TPA Frosted Doughnut 2%

CAP Glazed Doughnut 2%

CAP Raspberry v2 1,5%

TPA Raspberry sweet 0,5%

FA Custard 1%

FA Torrone 0,75%

FA Meringue 2%

FA Marshmallow 1%

CAP Super Sweet 0,75%

TPA Acetyl Pyrazine 5 PG 1%

3. Shake well and place your bottle of e-liquid in a dark place for 21 days. Enjoy vaping your new e-juice!

CHOCOLATE CHIP COOKIE DOUGH CHEESECAKE

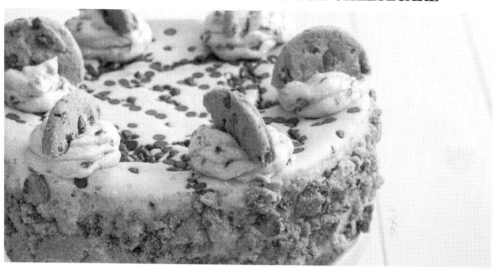

1. Grab your nic base. We recommend you use 70/30 VG/PG.

2. Add these flavours, and shake them well before mixing:

FA Cookie 2%

CAP Sugar Cookie 3%

FA Chocolate 1,5%

FA Cocoa 0,5%

CAP NY Cheesecake 4%

FA Custard 2%

FA Marshmallow 1%

CAP Super Sweet 0,75%

TPA Acetyl Pyrazine 5 PG 1%

3. Shake well and place your bottle of e-liquid in a dark place for 21-28 days. Enjoy vaping your new e-juice!

CARAMEL CHEESECAKE WITH MAPLE SYRUP

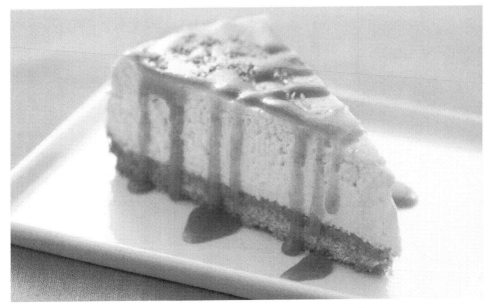

1. Grab your nic base. We recommend you use 70/30 VG/PG.

2. Add these flavours, and shake them well before mixing:

CAP NY Cheesecake 6%

CAP Golden Butter 0,5%

CAP Vanilla Custard 1%

FW Graham Cracker 1%

TPA Malted Milk 0,5%

FA Butterscotch 0,5%

FA Maple Syrup 0,25%

FA Marshmallow 1%

TPA Acetyl Pyrazine 5 PG 1%

3. Shake well and place your bottle of e-liquid in a dark place for 28 days. Enjoy vaping your new e-juice!

OREO CHEESECAKE

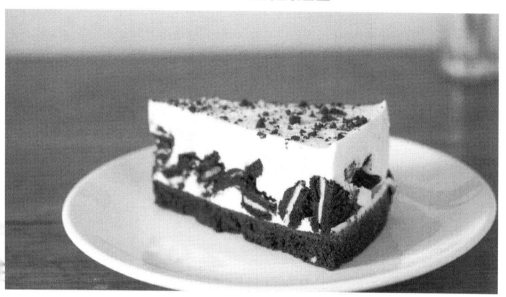

1. Grab your nic base. We recommend you use 70/30 VG/PG.

2. Add these flavours, and shake them well before mixing:

FW Cookies and Cream 7%

CAP Creamy Yogurt 2%

CAP NY Cheesecake 4%

FA Marshmallow 1%

TPA Acetyl Pyrazine 5 PG 1%

3. Shake well and place your bottle of e-liquid in a dark place for 21 days. Enjoy vaping your new e-juice!

PUMPKIN SPICE CHEESECAKE

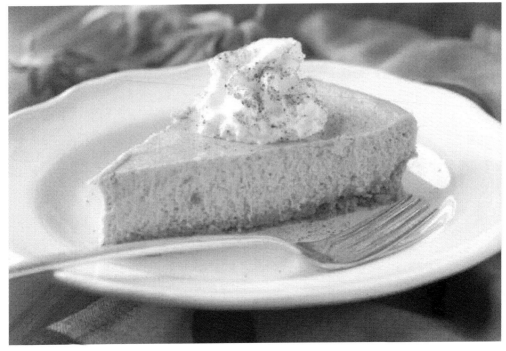

1. Grab your nic base. We recommend you use 70/30 VG/PG.

2. Add these flavours, and shake them well before mixing:

CAP NY Cheesecake 6%

CAP Vanilla Custard 1%

CAP Golden Butter 0,5%

FW Graham Cracker 1%

TPA Pumpkin Spice 3%

CAP French Vanilla 0,5%

FA Cinnamon Ceylon 0,5%

FA Marshmallow 1%

CAP Super Sweet 0,75%

TPA Acetyl Pyrazine 5 PG 1%

3. Shake well and place your bottle of e-liquid in a dark place for 21 days. Enjoy vaping your new e-juice!

TIRAMISU CHEESECAKE [OPEN RECIPE]

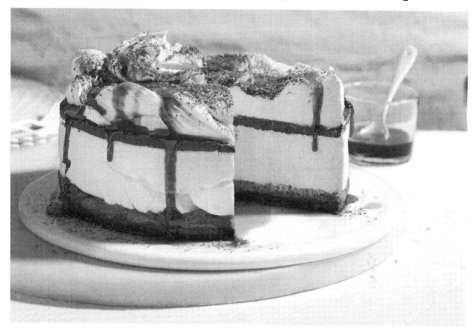

1. Grab your nic base. We recommend you use 70/30 VG/PG.

2. Add these flavours, and shake them well before mixing:

CAP Chocolate Fudge Brownie 4%

TPA Cheesecake Graham Crust 3%

CAP NY Cheesecake 2%

FA Tiramisu 1,25%

FA Fresh Cream 1%

FA Jamaican Rum 1%

CAP Vanilla Custard 2%

FA Marshmallow 1%

CAP Super Sweet 0,75%

TPA Acetyl Pyrazine 5 PG 1%

3. Shake well and place your bottle of e-liquid in a dark place for 21 days. Enjoy vaping your new e-juice!

PINEAPPLE, RASPBERRY & PASSIONFRUIT CHEESECAKE

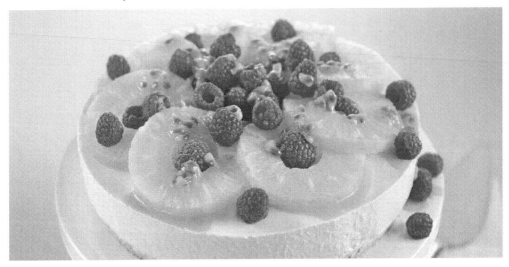

1. Grab your nic base. We recommend you use 70/30 VG/PG.

2. Add these flavours, and shake them well before mixing:

CAP NY Cheesecake 6%

FA Custard 2%

FW Graham Cracker 1%

TPA Passion Fruit 2%

FA Lemon Sicily 1%

CAP Raspberry v2 1,5%

TPA Raspberry sweet 0,5%

CAP Golden Pineapple 5%

TPA Acetyl Pyrazine 5 PG 1%

CAP Super Sweet 0,5%

3. Shake well and place your bottle of e-liquid in a dark place for 21 days. Enjoy vaping your new e-juice!

PISTACHIO CAKE

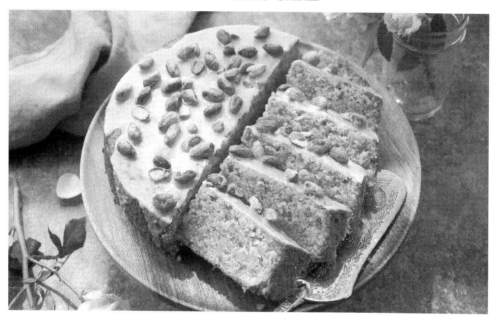

1. Grab your nic base. We recommend you use 70/30 VG/PG.

2. Add these flavours, and shake them well before mixing:

TPA Pistachio 8%

CAP NY Cheesecake 4%

FA Cookie 1%

TPA Graham Cracker 2%

TPA Coconut Extra 0,25%

FA Almond 1%

CAP Super Sweet 0,75%

TPA Acetyl Pyrazine 5 PG 1%

3. Shake well and place your bottle of e-liquid in a dark place for 21 days. Enjoy vaping your new e-juice!

LEMON CHEESECAKE

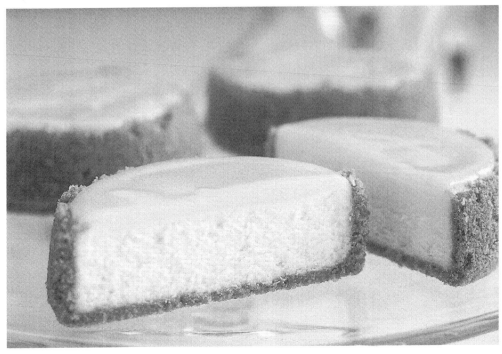

1. Grab your nic base. We recommend you use 70/30 VG/PG.

2. Add these flavours, and shake them well before mixing:

CAP Lemon Meringue Pie v1 6%

CAP New York Cheesecake 4%

TPA Cheesecake (Graham Crust) 2%

FA Vienna Cream 0.5%

FA Fresh Cream 0.5%

CAP French Vanilla 0,5%

TPA Acetyl Pyrazine 5 PG 1%

CAP Super Sweet 0,75%

3. Shake well and place your bottle of e-liquid in a dark place for 21 days. Enjoy vaping your new e-juice!

MOM'S APPLE FRITTERS

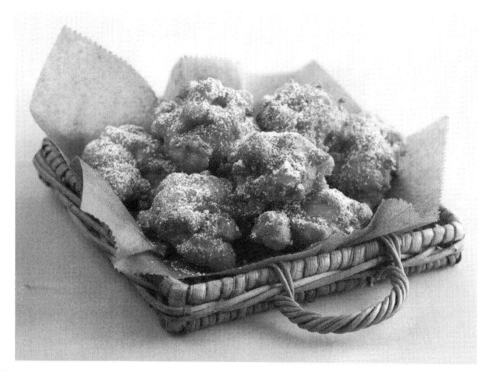

1. **Grab your nic base. We recommend you use 70/30 VG/PG.**

2. **Add these flavours, and shake them well before mixing:**

TPA Bavarian Cream 3%

FA Apple Pie 4%

FA Almond 0,5%

FA Joy 0,5%

CAP Cinnamon Danish Swirl v2 3%

FA Meringue 2%

FA Torrone 0,75%

FA Cardamom 0,5%

CAP Super Sweet 0,75%

TPA Acetyl Pyrazine 5 PG 1%

3. **Shake well and place your bottle of e-liquid in a dark place for 21 days. Enjoy vaping your new e-juice!**

BAKED APPLES WITH CINNAMON AND HONEY

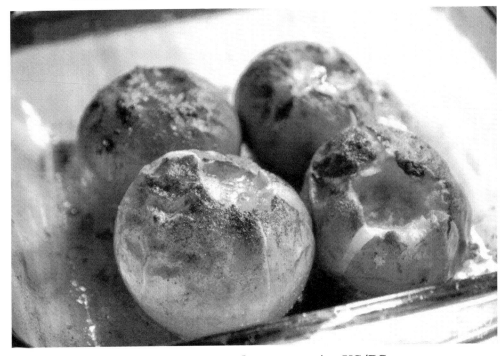

1. Grab your nic base. We recommend you use 70/30 VG/PG.

2. Add these flavours, and shake them well before mixing:

CAP Cinnamon Danish Swirl v1 1%

FA Maple Syrup 0,25%

FA Liquid Amber 0,5%

FA Brandy 0,5%

FA Butterscotch 0,5%

FA Cinnamon Ceylon 0,25%

TPA Brown Sugar 0,25%

FA Marshmallow 1%

FW Green Apple 6% or CAP Double Apple 5%

TPA Acetyl Pyrazine 5 PG 1%

3. Shake well and place your bottle of e-liquid in a dark place for 21 - 28 days. Enjoy vaping your new e-juice!

CHOCOLATE BANANA COFFEE CAKE

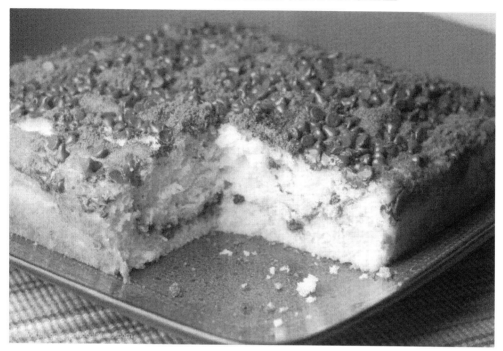

1. Grab your nic base. We recommend you use 70/30 VG/PG.

2. Add these flavours, and shake them well before mixing:

TPA Banana Nut Bread 5%

CAP Cake Batter 2%

FA Cookie 0.25%

FA Irish Cream 3%

FA Cream Fresh 0.5%

FA Vienna Cream 0.5%

FA Marshmallow 1%

CAP Super Sweet 0,75%

TPA Acetyl Pyrazine 5 PG 1%

3. Shake well and place your bottle of e-liquid in a dark place for 21 days. Enjoy vaping your new e-juice!

TIRAMISU CAKE

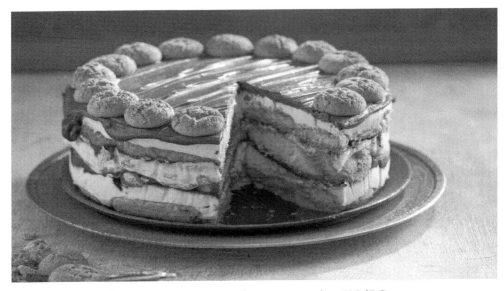

1. Grab your nic base. We recommend you use 70/30 VG/PG.

2. Add these flavours, and shake them well before mixing:

FW Cake Batter Dip 6%

FA Tiramisu 1,5%

FA Catalan Cream 3%

FA Cream Fresh 1%

FA Vienna Cream 2%

FA Custard 2%

FA Marshmallow 1%

CAP Super Sweet 0,75%

TPA Acetyl Pyrazine 5 PG 1%

3. Shake well and place your bottle of e-liquid in a dark place for 21 days. Enjoy vaping your new e-juice!

CARIBBEAN RUM CAKE

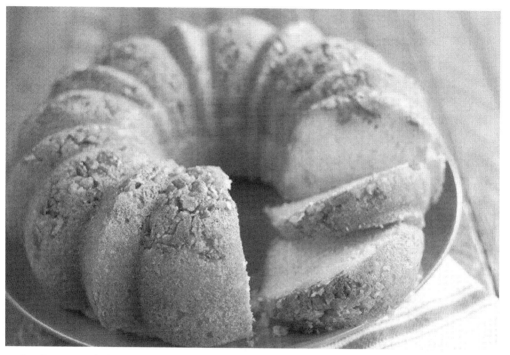

1. Grab your nic base. We recommend you use 70/30 VG/PG.

2. Add these flavours, and shake them well before mixing:

FA Jamaican Rum 3%

CAP Yellow Cake 2%

FA Custard 2%

FW Yellow Cake 1,5%

FA Cookie 1%

FW Graham Cracker 2%

FA Maple Syrup 0,25%

TPA Acetyl Pyrazine 5 PG 1%

3. Shake well and place your bottle of e-liquid in a dark place for 21 days.
Enjoy vaping your new e-juice!

GLAZED PEACH PIE

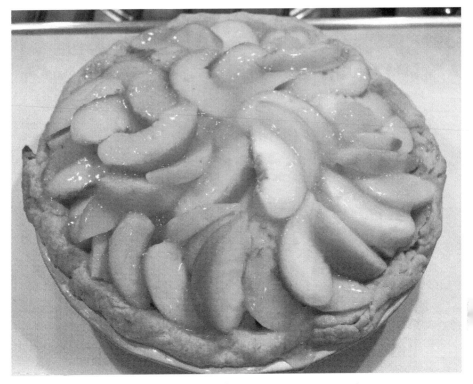

1. Grab your nic base. We recommend you use 70/30 VG/PG.

2. Add these flavours, and shake them well before mixing:

FA Apple Pie 2%

FA Cookie 1%

CAP Cinnamon Danish Swirl v1 3%

FA White Peach 0,75%

TPA Peach (Juicy) 3%

FA Liquid Amber 0,5%

FA Custard 1%

FA Caramel 0,5%

FA Maple Syrup 0,25%

TPA Acetyl Pyrazine 5 PG 1%

3. Shake well and place your bottle of e-liquid in a dark place for 21 days. Enjoy vaping your new e-juice!

BAKED APPLES WITH RUM-CARAMEL SAUCE

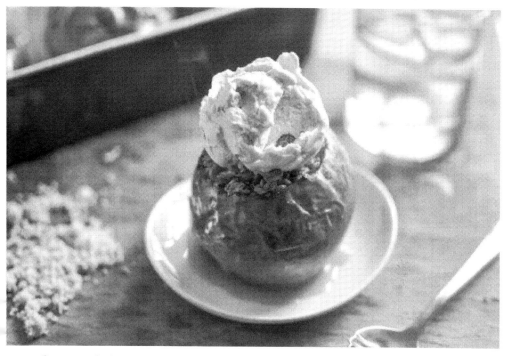

1. Grab your nic base. We recommend you use 70/30 VG/PG.

2. Add these flavours, and shake them well before mixing:

CAP Cinnamon Danish Swirl v1 1%

FA Maple Syrup 0,25%

FA Liquid Amber 0,5%

FA Custard 2%

FA Jamaican Rum 2%

FA Cinnamon Ceylon 0,25%

TPA Brown Sugar 0,25%

FA Marshmallow 1%

FW Green Apple 6% or CAP Double Apple 5%

TPA Acetyl Pyrazine 5 PG 1%

3. Shake well and place your bottle of e-liquid in a dark place for 21 days. Enjoy vaping your new e-juice!

LEMON PIE WITH RASPBERRY JAM

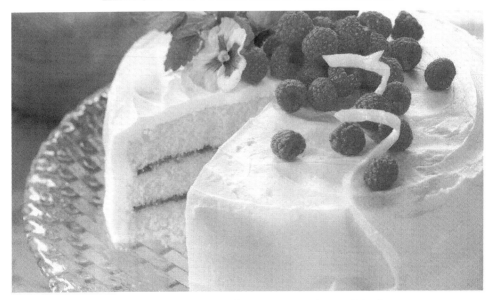

1. Grab your nic base. We recommend you use 70/30 VG/PG.

2. Add these flavours, and shake them well bcfore mixing:

CAP Lemon Meringue Pie v1 6%

CAP Yellow Cake 2%

FA Custard 2%

FW Graham Cracker 1%

CAP Raspberry v2 1,5%

TPA Raspberry sweet 0,5%

FA Marshmallow 1%

CAP Super Sweet 0,75%

TPA Acetyl Pyrazine 5 PG 1%

3. Shake well and place your bottle of e-liquid in a dark place for 21 days. Enjoy vaping your new e-juice!

BELGIAN WAFFLES WITH MAPLE SYRUP

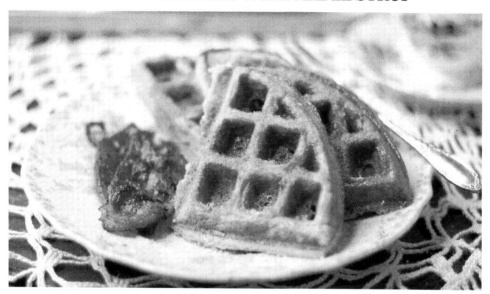

1. Grab your nic base. We recommend you use 70/30 VG/PG.

2. Add these flavours, and shake them well before mixing:

TPA Waffle (Belgian) 8%

FA Catalan Cream 3%

FA Cream Fresh 1%

FA Vienna Cream 2%

FA Marshmallow 1%

FA Maple Syrup 0,25%

FA Cardamom 0,5%

TPA Acetyl Pyrazine 5 PG 1%

3. Shake well and place your bottle of e-liquid in a dark place for 21 days. Enjoy vaping your new e-juice!

BLUEBERRY CUPCAKE

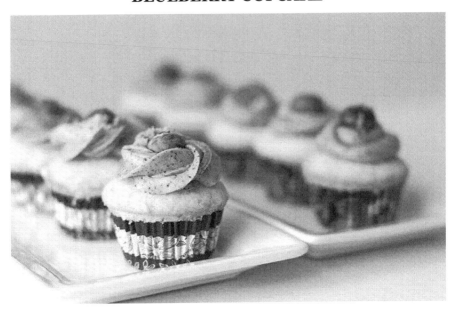

1. Grab your nic base. We recommend you use 70/30 VG/PG.

2. Add these flavours, and shake them well before mixing:

FW Yellow Cake 2%

CAP Vanilla Cupcake 6%

TPA Blueberry Extra 4%

TPA Blueberry Wild 3%

FA Torrone 0,75%

CAP Super sweet 0,5%

TPA Acetyl Pyrazine 5 PG 1%

3. Shake well and place your bottle of e-liquid in a dark place for 21 days. Enjoy vaping your new e-juice!

CITRUS PIE

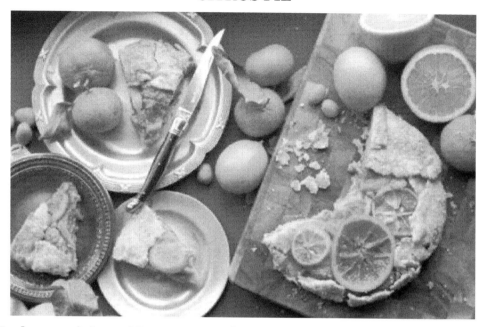

1. Grab your nic base. We recommend you use 70/30 VG/PG.

2. Add these flavours, and shake them well before mixing:

CAP Lemon Meringue Pie v1 6%

FA Cookie 1%

TPA Graham Cracker 2%

CAP Sweet Tangerine 6,5%

FA Catalan Cream 3%

FA Cardamom 0,5%

FA Bergamot 0,5%

FA Marshmallow 1%

CAP Super Sweet 0,75%

TPA Acetyl Pyrazine 5 PG 1%

3. Shake well and place your bottle of e-liquid in a dark place for 21 days. Enjoy vaping your new e-juice!

CHOCOLATE CAKE WITH BLUE CURRANT AND RUM

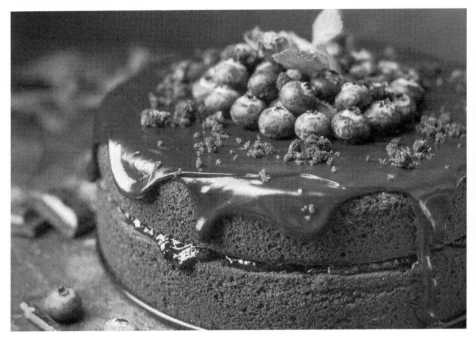

1. Grab your nic base. We recommend you use 70/30 VG/PG.

2. Add these flavours, and shake them well before mixing:

CAP Chocolate Fudge Brownie 5%

CAP Cake Batter 2%

FA Custard 2%

FA Lemon Sicily 0.3%

FA Jamaican Rum 1,5%

TPA Blueberry Extra 4%

TPA Blueberry Wild 3%

TPA Bavarian Cream 2%

CAP Super Sweet 0,75%

TPA Acetyl Pyrazine 5 PG 1%

3. Shake well and place your bottle of e-liquid in a dark place for 21 days. Enjoy vaping your new e-juice!

BISCOTTI GELATO

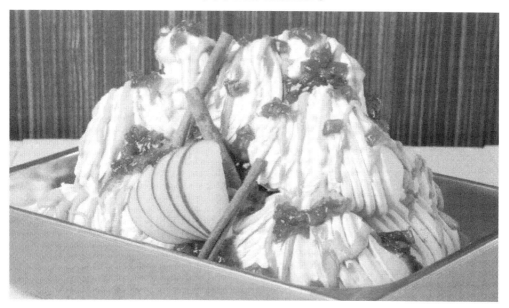

1. Grab your nic base. We recommend you use 70/30 VG/PG.

2. Add these flavours, and shake them well before mixing:

FA Cookie 3%

FA Cinnamon Ceylon 0,5%

FA Catalan Cream 3%

FA Cream Fresh 1%

FA Vienna Cream 2%

FA Custard 2%

FA Marshmallow 1%

CAP Super Sweet 0,75%

TPA Acetyl Pyrazine 5 PG 1%

Shake well and place your bottle of e-liquid in a dark place for 21 days. Enjoy vaping your new e-juice!

GREEK YOGURT WHIPPED CREAM

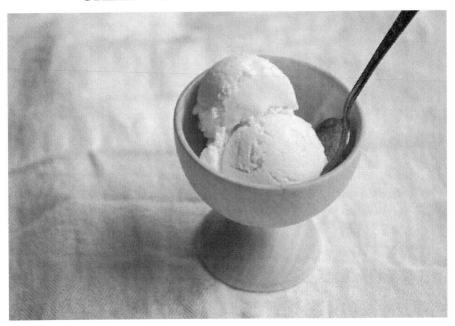

1. Grab your nic base. We recommend you use 70/30 VG/PG.

2. Add these flavours, and shake them well before mixing:

CAP Cream Yogurt 2%

FA Catalan Cream 3%

FA Cream Fresh 1%

FA Vienna Cream 2%

FA Custard 2%

FA Marshmallow 1%

CAP Super Sweet 0,75%

TPA Greek Yogurt 2%

CAP French Vanilla 0,5%

3. Shake well and place your bottle of e-liquid in a dark place for 21 days. Enjoy vaping your new e-juice!

OLD SCHOOL

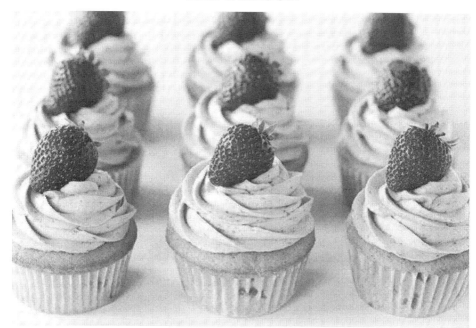

1. Grab your nic base. We recommend you use 70/30 VG/PG.

2. Add these flavours, and shake them well before mixing:

TPA Strawberry Ripe 2%

CAP Sweet Strawberry 4%

CAP Vanilla Cupcake 5%

FA Cream Fresh 1%

FA Vienna Cream 2%

FA Custard 2%

FA Marshmallow 1%

CAP Super Sweet 0,75%

TPA Acetyl Pyrazine 5 PG 1%

3. Shake well and place your bottle of e-liquid in a dark place for 21 days. Enjoy vaping your new e-juice!

GRAPEFRUIT GELATO

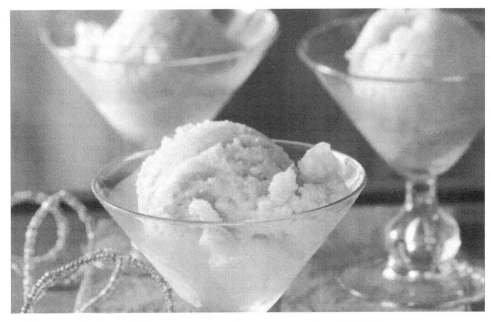

1. Grab your nic base. We recommend you use 70/30 VG/PG.

2. Add these flavours, and shake them well before mixing:

FA Grapefruit 4%

FA Catalan Cream 3%

FA Cream Fresh 1%

FA Vienna Cream 2%

FA Custard 2%

FA Marshmallow 1%

CAP Super Sweet 0,75%

FA Polar Blast 1% or TPA Koolada 1%

3. Shake well and place your bottle of e-liquid in a dark place for 21 days. Enjoy vaping your new e-juice!

POMEGRANATE GELATO

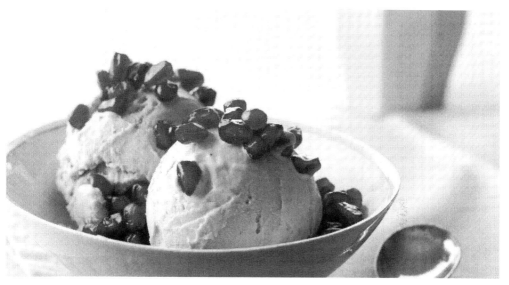

1. Grab your nic base. We recommend you use 70/30 VG/PG.

2. Add these flavours, and shake them well before mixing:

FA Pomegranate 1,5%

TPA Dragonfruit 0,75%

TPA Taro 2%

FA Cream Fresh 1%

FA Vienna Cream 2%

FA Custard 3%

FA Marshmallow 1%

FA Polar Blast 1% or TPA Koolada 1%

3. Shake well and place your bottle of e-liquid in a dark place for 21 days. Enjoy vaping your new e-juice!

BLUEBERRY GELATO

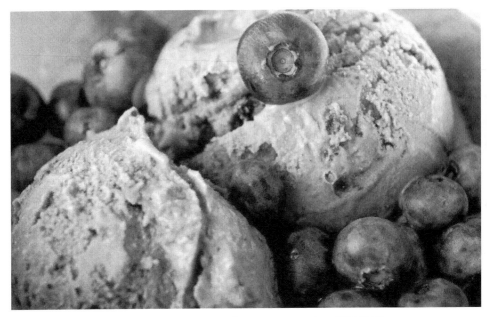

1. Grab your nic base. We recommend you use 70/30 VG/PG.

2. Add these flavours, and shake them well before mixing:

TPA Blueberry Extra 4%

TPA Blueberry Wild 3%

FA Catalan Cream 3%

FA Cream Fresh 1%

FA Vienna Cream 2%

FA Custard 2%

FA Marshmallow 1%

CAP Super Sweet 0,75%

FA Polar Blast 1% or TPA Koolada 1%

3. Shake well and place your bottle of e-liquid in a dark place for 21 days. Enjoy vaping your new e-juice!

STRAWBERRY GELATO

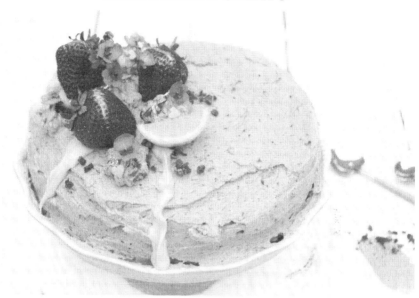

1. Grab your nic base. We recommend you use 70/30 VG/PG.

2. Add these flavours, and shake them well before mixing:

CAP Sweet Strawberry 3% or 4%, depending on your taste.

TPA Strawberry Ripe 2%

FA Catalan Cream 3%

FA Vienna Cream 2%

FA Custard 2%

FA Marshmallow 1%

CAP Super Sweet 0,75%

FA Polar Blast 1% or TPA Koolada 1%

3. Shake well and place your bottle of e-liquid in a dark place for 14 - 21 days. Enjoy vaping your new e-juice!

BANANA PUDDING

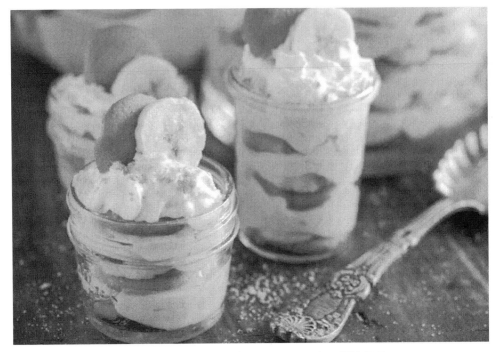

1. Grab your nic base. We recommend you use 70/30 VG/PG.

2. Add these flavours, and shake them well before mixing:

TPA Banana Cream 6%

CAP Vanilla Custard 2%

CAP Sugar Cookie 3,5%

CAP Golden Butter 0,5%

CAP Creamy Yogurt 2%

FA Marshmallow 1%

CAP Super Sweet 0,75%

CAP French Vanilla 0,5%

TPA Acetyl Pyrazine 5 PG 1%

3. Shake well and place your bottle of e-liquid in a dark place for 21 days. Enjoy vaping your new e-juice!

PEACHES AND ICE CREAM

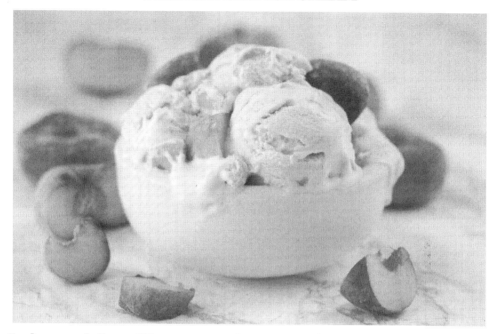

1. Grab your nic base. We recommend you use 70/30 VG/PG.

2. Add these flavours, and shake them well before mixing:

CAP Peaches and Cream 6%

TPA Dragonfruit 3%

FA Catalan Cream 3%

FA Cream Fresh 1%

FA Vienna Cream 2%

FA Custard 2%

FA Cardamom 0,5%

FA Marshmallow 1%

CAP Super Sweet 0,75%

3. Shake well and place your bottle of e-liquid in a dark place for 21 days. Enjoy vaping your new e-juice!

FRIED ICE CREAM

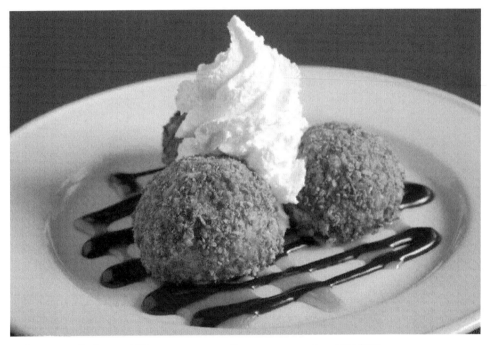

1. Grab your nic base. We recommend you use 70/30 VG/PG.

2. Add these flavours, and shake them well before mixing:

CAP Cereal 27 2%

CAP Sugar Cookie 3%

FA Catalan Cream 3%

FA Cream Fresh 1%

FA Vienna Cream 2%

FA Custard 2%

FA Marshmallow 1%

FA Maple Syrup 0,25%

TPA Acetyl Pyrazine 5 PG 1%

3. Shake well and place your bottle of e-liquid in a dark place for 21 days. Enjoy vaping your new e-juice!

RASPBERRY MUFFIN

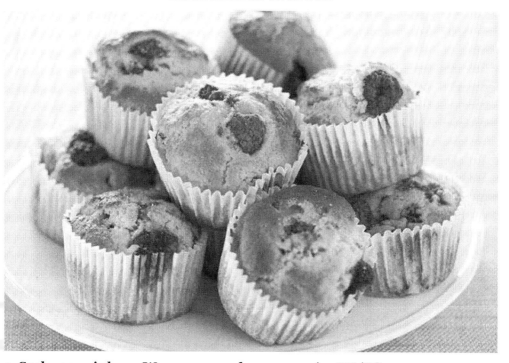

1. Grab your nic base. We recommend you use 70/30 VG/PG.

2. Add these flavours, and shake them well before mixing:

CAP Vanilla Cupcake 6%

CAP Cake Batter 2%

CAP Raspberry v2 1,5%

TPA Raspberry sweet 0,5%

FA Lemon Sicily 0,5%

CAP Super Sweet 0,5%

TPA Acetyl Pyrazine 5 PG 1%

3. Shake well and place your bottle of e-liquid in a dark place for 21 days. Enjoy vaping your new e-juice!

BANANA SPLIT

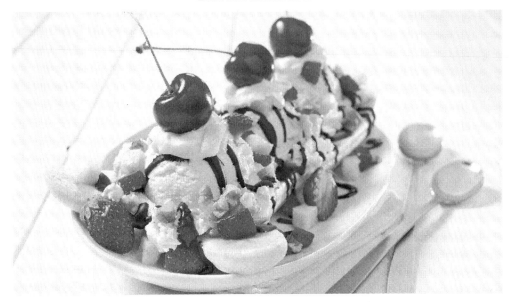

1. Grab your nic base. We recommend you use 70/30 VG/PG.

2. Add these flavours, and shake them well before mixing:

FW Beetle Juice 6%

TPA Dragonfruit 0,75%

TPA Banana Cream 6%

FA Custard 2%

FA Lemon Sicily 0,3%

FA Marshmallow 1%

CAP Super Sweet 0,5%

3. Shake well and place your bottle of e-liquid in a dark place for 28 days. Enjoy vaping your new e-juice!

CHAPTER 3: DRINK RECIPES

ORANGE SPICE TEA

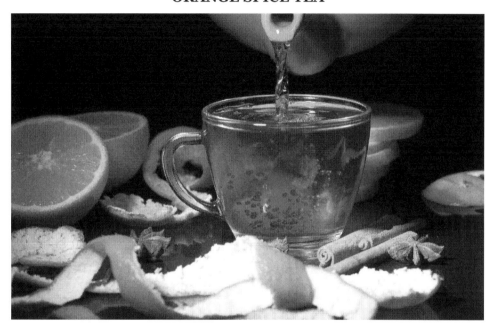

1. Grab your nic base. We recommend you use 70/30 VG/PG.

2. Add these flavours, and shake them well before mixing:

FW Blood Orange 4%

CAP Sweet Tea 5%

CAP Juicy Lemon 2%

FA Cinnamon Ceylon 0,25%

FA Bergamot 0,5%

3. Shake well and place your bottle of e-liquid in a dark place for 21 days. Enjoy vaping your new e-juice!

EARL GREY SPICE TEA

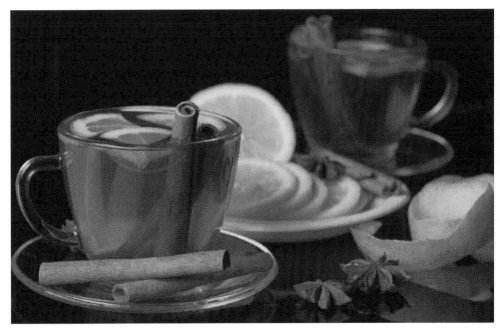

1. Grab your nic base. We recommend you use 70/30 VG/PG.

2. Add these flavours, and shake them well before mixing:

FA Black Tea 3,5%

CAP Juicy Lemon 2%

TPA Black Honey 1%

FA Cinnamon Ceylon 0,25%

FA Cardamom 0,5%

FA Bergamot 0,5%

FA Fresh Cream 1%

3. Shake well and place your bottle of e-liquid in a dark place for 21 days. Enjoy vaping your new e-juice!

SANGRIA COCKTAIL VAPE

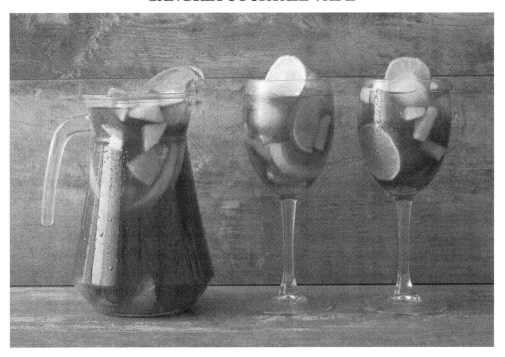

1. Grab your nic base. We recommend you use 70/30 VG/PG.

2. Add these flavours, and shake them well before mixing:

CAP Pink Lemonade 5%

FA Raspberry 1,5%

(Optional) FA Brandy 1%

TPA Dragonfruit 0,75%

FA Cardamom 0,5%

TPA Champagne 1% - fizzy effect.

CAP Lemon Lime 1% - fizzy effect.

FA Polar Blast 0,75% or TPA Koolada 0,75%

CAP Super Sweet 0,75%

3. Shake well and place your bottle of e-liquid in a dark place for 21 days. Enjoy vaping your new e-juice!

PUMPKIN SPICE LATTE

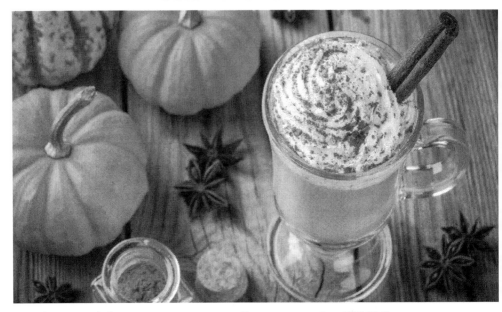

1. Grab your nic base. We recommend you use 70/30 VG/PG.

2. Add these flavours, and shake them well before mixing:

FW Pumpkin Spice 3% or TPA Pumpkin Spice 3%

(Optional) FA Anise 0,5%

FA Caramel 0,5%

FA Tiramisu 0,75%

FA Catalan Cream 3%

FA Cream Fresh 1%

FA Vienna Cream 2%

FA Custard 2%

FA Marshmallow 1%

3. Shake well and place your bottle of e-liquid in a dark place for 28 days. Enjoy vaping your new e-juice!

PUMPKIN SPICE LATTE REMIX

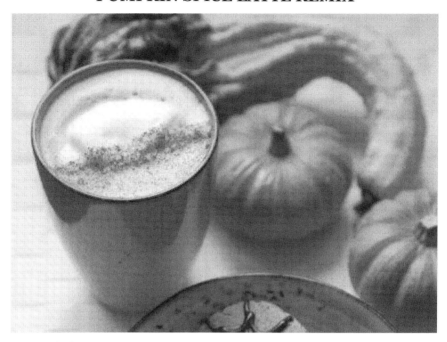

1. Grab your nic base. We recommend you use 70/30 VG/PG.

2. Add these flavours, and shake them well before mixing:

FW Pumpkin Spice 2% or TPA Pumpkin Spice 2%

CAP Hot Cocoa 5,5%

FA Tiramisu 0,75%

FA Vienna Cream 2%

FA Caramel 1%

FA Dark Bean 0,5%

FA Marshmallow 1%

CAP Super Sweet 0,75%

TPA Acetyl Pyrazine 5 PG 1%

CAP French Vanilla 1%

3. Shake well and place your bottle of e-liquid in a dark place for 28 days.
Enjoy vaping your new e-juice!

IRISH CREAM COFFEE

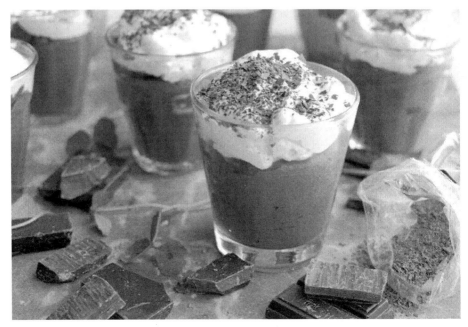

1. Grab your nic base. We recommend you use 70/30 VG/PG.

2. Add these flavours, and shake them well before mixing:

FA Irish cream 3%

FA Fresh Cream 3%

FA Vienna Cream 2%

FA Chocolate 1,5%

FA Cocoa 0,5%

FA Caramel 0,5%

FA Marshmallow 1%

CAP Super Sweet 0,75%

TPA Acetyl Pyrazine 5 PG 1%

3. Shake well and place your bottle of e-liquid in a dark place for 28 days. Enjoy vaping your new e-juice!

SPICED-RUM COFFEE WITH BUTTERSCOTCH WHIPPED CREAM (FOR HIM)

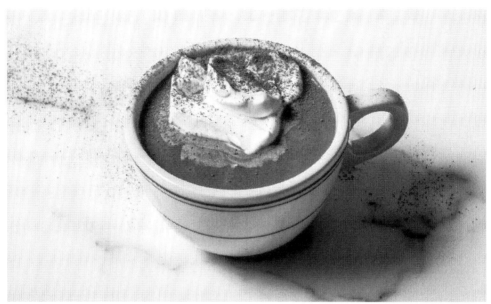

1. Grab your nic base. We recommend you use 70/30 VG/PG.

2. Add these flavours, and shake them well before mixing:

FA Butterscotch 2%

FA Jamaican Rum 1%

FA Irish Cream 2%

FA Dark Bean (Espresso) 2%

FA Catalan Cream 3%

FA Cream Fresh 1%

FA Vienna Cream 2%

FA Custard 2%

FA Marshmallow 1%

CAP Super Sweet 0,75%

TPA Acetyl Pyrazine 5 PG 1%

3. Shake well and place your bottle of e-liquid in a dark place for 28 days. Enjoy vaping your new e-juice!

CREAMY AMARETTO LIQUEUR COFFEE (FOR HER)

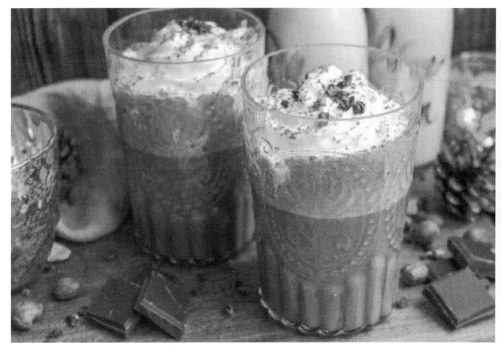

1. Grab your nic base. We recommend you use 70/30 VG/PG.

2. Add these flavours, and shake them well before mixing:

FA Vanilla Tahiti 1,25%

FA Marzipan 0,75%

FA Vanilla Bourbon 0,75%

FA Caramel 0,75%

FA Fresh Cream 1,5%

FA Tiramisu 0,75%

FA Dark Bean 1%

FA Marshmallow 1%

CAP Super Sweet 0,75%

TPA Acetyl Pyrazine 5 PG 1%

3. Shake well and place your bottle of e-liquid in a dark place for 21 days. Enjoy vaping your new e-juice!

PEANUT BUTTER HOT CHOCOLATE

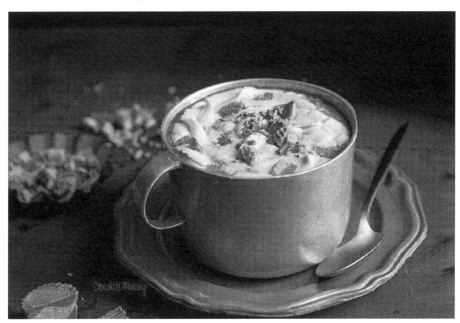

1. Grab your nic base. We recommend you use 70/30 VG/PG.

2. Add these flavours, and shake them well before mixing:

FA Irish Cream 3% or CAP Hot Cocoa 5,5%

CAP Peanut Butter v1 1%

TPA Peanut Butter 6,5%

FA Catalan Cream 3%

FA Cream Fresh 1%

FA Vienna Cream 2%

FA Custard 2%

FA Marshmallow 1%

CAP Super Sweet 0,75%

TPA Acetyl Pyrazine 5 PG 1%

3. Shake well and place your bottle of e-liquid in a dark place for at least 21 days. Enjoy vaping your new e-juice!

NUTELLA FRANGELICO HOT CHOCOLATE

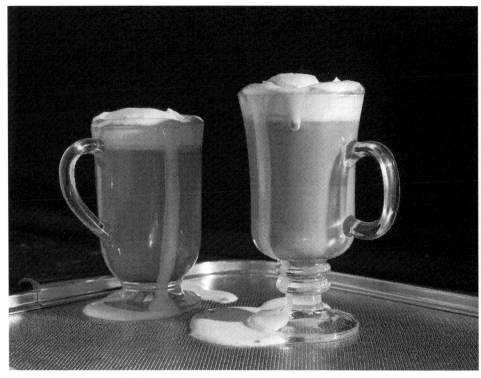

1. Grab your nic base. We recommend you use 70/30 VG/PG.

2. Add these flavours, and shake them well before mixing:

FA Irish Cream 3%

FA Hazelnut 1,5%

FA Brandy 0,5%

FA Cocoa 1,5%

FA Cream Fresh 1%

FA Vienna Cream 2%

FA Marshmallow 1%

CAP Super Sweet 0,75%

TPA Acetyl Pyrazine 5 PG 1%

3. Shake well and place your bottle of e-liquid in a dark place for 28 days. Enjoy vaping your new e-juice!

HOMEMADE BUTTERBEER (VERSION 6)

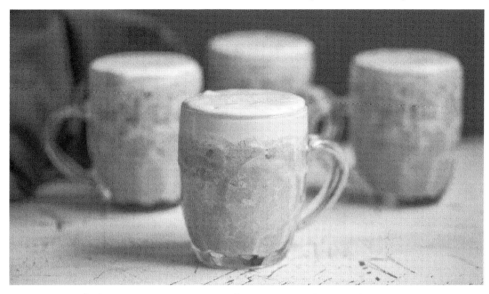

1. Grab your nic base. We recommend you use 70/30 VG/PG.

2. Add these flavours, and shake them well before mixing:

FA Jamaican Rum 2%

FA Vienna Cream 2%

FW Butterscotch Ripple 2%

FA Caramel 1%

CAP Golden Butter 0,5%

TPA Whipped Cream 2%

FA Marshmallow 1%

CAP Super Sweet 0,75%

3. Shake well and place your bottle of e-liquid in a dark place for 28 days. Enjoy vaping your new e-juice!

BANANA MILKSHAKE WITH CARAMEL

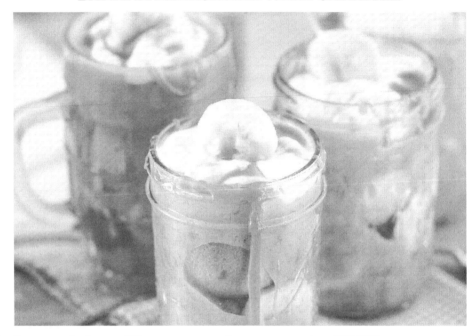

1. Grab your nic base. We recommend you use 70/30 VG/PG.

2. Add these flavours, and shake them well before mixing:

TPA Banana Cream 5%

TPA Malted Milk 0,5%

FA Butterscotch 0,5%

FA Caramel 1%

FA Cream Fresh 1%

FA Vienna Cream 2%

FA Custard 2%

FA Marshmallow 1%

CAP Super Sweet 0,75%

TPA Acetyl Pyrazine 5 PG 0,5%

3. Shake well and place your bottle of e-liquid in a dark place for 28 days. Enjoy vaping your new e-juice!

AUTHENTIC HORCHATA

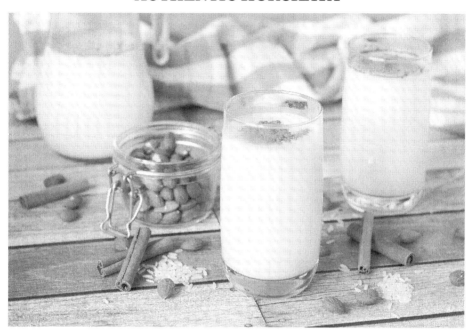

1. Grab your nic base. We recommend you use 70/30 VG/PG.

2. Add these flavours, and shake them well before mixing:

CAP Horchata 5%

CAP Hot Cocoa 5,5%

FA Catalan Cream 3%

FA Cream Fresh 1%

FA Vienna Cream 2%

FA Custard 2%

FA Marshmallow 1%

CAP Super Sweet 0,75%

TPA Acetyl Pyrazine 5 PG 0,5%

3. Shake well and place your bottle of e-liquid in a dark place for 28 days. Enjoy vaping your new e-juice!

JASMINE GREEN TEA

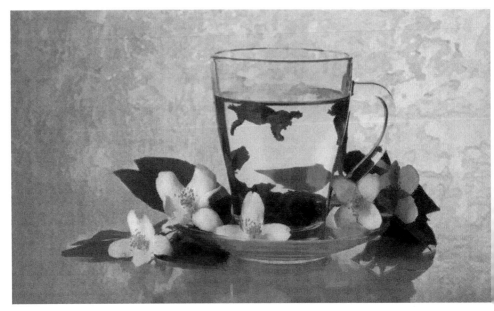

1. Grab your nic base. We recommend you use 70/30 VG/PG.

2. Add these flavours, and shake them well before mixing:

CAP Sweet Tea 5%

CAP Juicy Lemon 1,5%

TPA Green Tea 3,5%

FA Jasmine 1,5%

FA Cardamom 0,5%

CAP Super Sweet 0,75%

3. Shake well and place your bottle of e-liquid in a dark place for 21 days. Enjoy vaping your new e-juice!

RASPBERRY LEMONADE (TASTE LIKE REMIX OF ZENITH ORION)

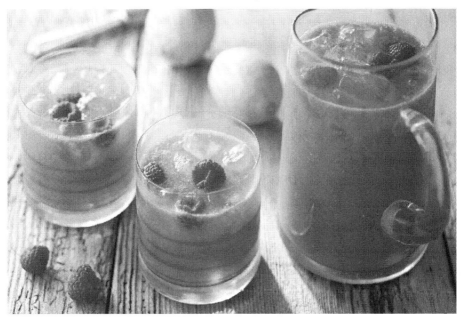

1. Grab your nic base. We recommend you use 70/30 VG/PG.

2. Add these flavours, and shake them well before mixing:

CAP Pink Lemonade 5%

TPA Champagne 1%

CAP Lemon Lime 1%

FA Raspberry 2% or CAP Raspberry v2 2%

CAP Juicy Lemon 2%

FA Polar Blast 0,75% or TPA Koolada 0,75%

3. Shake well and place your bottle of e-liquid in a dark place for 21 days. Enjoy vaping your new e-juice!

CITRUS CREAM SODA

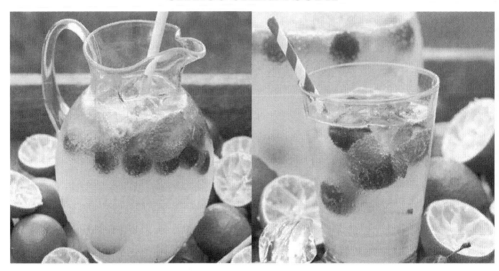

1. Grab your nic base. We recommend you use 70/30 VG/PG.

2. Add these flavours, and shake them well before mixing:

FA Oba Oba 5%

CAP Harvest Berry 2%

TPA Citrus Punch 6,5%

FA Lemon Sicily 0,5%

TPA Champagne 1%

3. Shake well and place your bottle of e-liquid in a dark place for 14 days. Enjoy vaping your new e-juice!

PINEAPPLE CREAM SODA

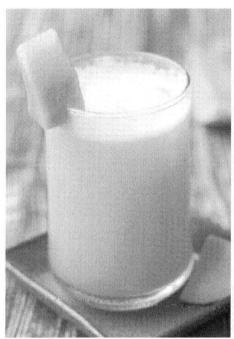 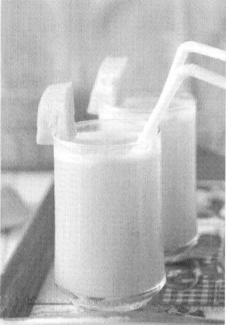

1. Grab your nic base. We recommend you use 70/30 VG/PG.

2. Add these flavours, and shake them well before mixing:

CAP Golden Pineapple 5%

FA Mandarin 4%

FA Oba Oba 5%

TPA Champagne 1%

FA Lemon Sicily 0,5%

TPA Dragonfruit 0,75%

3. Shake well and place your bottle of e-liquid in a dark place for 28 days. Enjoy vaping your new e-juice!

BUBBLY CREAM SODA

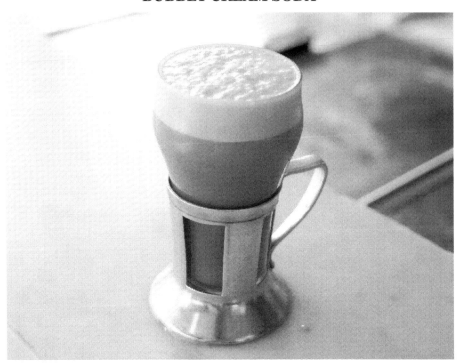

1. Grab your nic base. We recommend you use 70/30 VG/PG.

2. Add these flavours, and shake them well before mixing:

FA Oba Oba 5%

TPA Whipped Cream 2%

CAP Lemon Lime 1%

TPA Champagne 1,5%

3. Shake well and place your bottle of e-liquid in a dark place for 14 days. Enjoy vaping your new e-juice!

CHAPTER 4: ALCOHOL-INSPIRED E-JUICES

APPLE WHISKY "FAMOUS JOY"

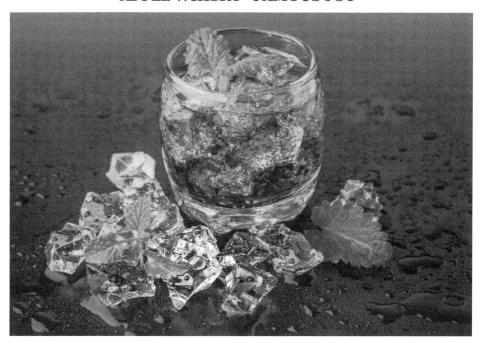

1. Grab your nic base. We recommend you use 70/30 VG/PG.

2. Add these flavours, and shake them well before mixing:

FA Whisky 1,5%

TPA Apple 6%

FA Oak Wood 1,5%

FA Liquid Amber 1% or 2%, depending on your taste.

CAP Lemon Lime 2%

FA Maple Syrup 0,25%

FA Polar Blast 0,5% or TPA Koolada 0,5%

FA Cinnamon Ceylon 0,25%

3. Shake well and place your bottle of e-liquid in a dark place from 25 to 40 days. Enjoy vaping your new e-juice!

PEACH BOURBON
(OUR MOST UNIQUE RECIPE)

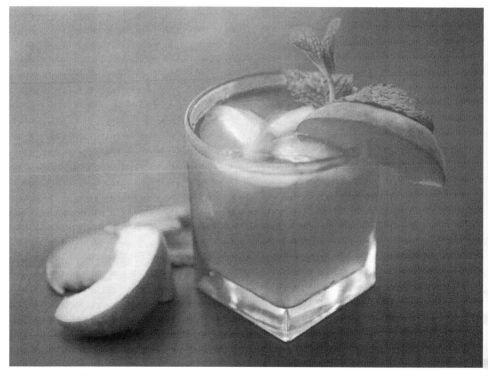

1. Grab your nic base. We recommend you use 70/30 VG/PG.

2. Add these flavours, and shake them well before mixing:

TPA Kentucky Bourbon 2% or FA Whisky 1,5%

FA White Peach 0,75%

TPA Peach (Juicy) 3%

TPA Red Oak 1,5%

FA Oak Wood 0,5%

FA Liquid Amber 1%

FA Maple Syrup 0,25%

FA Cinnamon Ceylon 0,25%

3. Shake well and place your bottle of e-liquid in a dark place from 25 to 40 days. Enjoy vaping your new e-juice!

OAK WOOD RUM AND COLA

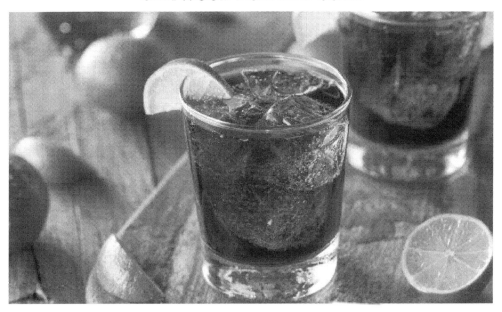

1. Grab your nic base. We recommend you use 70/30 VG/PG.

2. Add these flavours, and shake them well before mixing:

FA Jamaican Rum 3% or 4%. Depending on your taste.

FA Oak Wood 1%

FA Cola 4%

FA Black Cherry 2%

CAP Lemon Lime 2%

TPA Brown Sugar 0,25%

FA Polar Blast 0,5% or TPA Koolada 0,5%

3. Shake well and place your bottle of e-liquid in a dark place from 25 to 40 days. Enjoy vaping your new e-juice!

CASTLE LONG REMIX

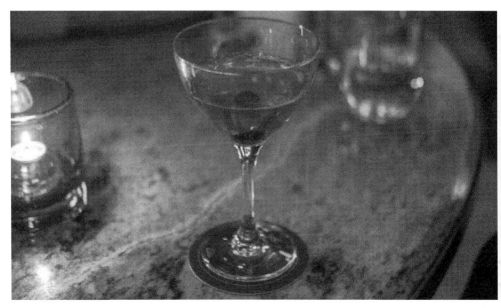

1. Grab your nic base. We recommend you use 70/30 VG/PG.

2. Add these flavours, and shake them well before mixing:

FA Jamaican Rum 4%

FA Vanilla Bourbon 2%

TPA Kentucky Bourbon 4%

TPA Red Oak 1,5%

FA Oak Wood 0,5%

CAP Juicy Lemon 2%

TPA Toasted Almond 2%

TPA Brown Sugar 0,5% or FA Maple Syrup 0,25%

3. Shake well and place your bottle of e-liquid in a dark place from 25 to 40 days. Enjoy vaping your new e-juice!

KENTUCKY BOURBON WITH SPICE APPLE JUICE

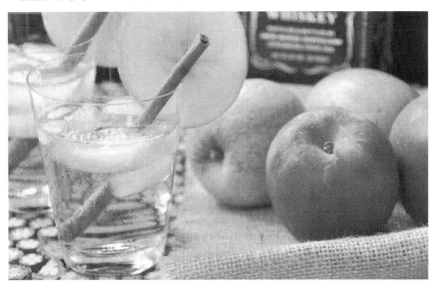

1. Grab your nic base. We recommend you use 70/30 VG/PG.

2. Add these flavours, and shake them well before mixing:

TPA Kentucky Bourbon 3% or 4%, depending on your taste

(Optional) TPA Black Honey 1%

TPA Apple 6%

FA Oak Wood 1,5%

TPA Brown Sugar 0,25%

CAP Juicy Lemon 2%

FA Cinnamon Ceylon 0,5%

FA Maple Syrup 0,25%

3. Shake well and place your bottle of e-liquid in a dark place from 25 to 40 days. Enjoy vaping your new e-juice!

PEAR CIDER

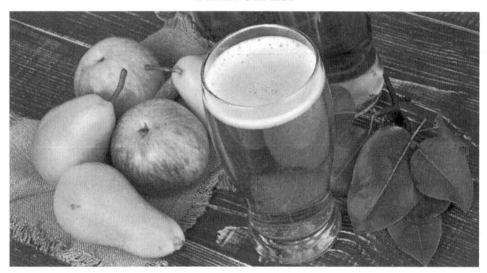

1. Grab your nic base. We recommend you use 70/30 VG/PG.

2. Add these flavours, and shake them well before mixing:

TPA Dragonfruit 0,75%

TPA Apple 6%

TPA Pear 5,5%

FA Liquid Amber 1,0%

FA Oakwood 1%

CAP French Vanilla 1,0%

FA Cinnamon Ceylon 0,25%

TPA Champagne 1% - fizzy effect.

3. Shake well and place your bottle of e-liquid in a dark place for 21 days. Enjoy vaping your new e-juice!

CHAPTER 5: SPECIAL FRUIT RECIPES

TROPICAL ISLAND

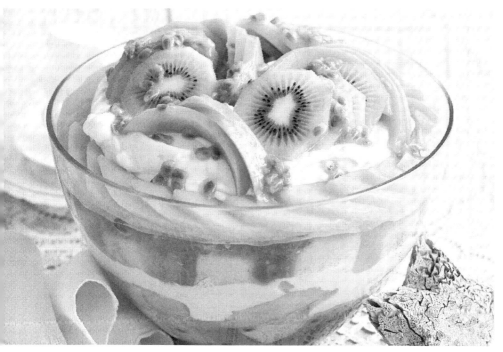

1. Grab your nic base. We recommend you use 70/30 VG/PG.

2. Add these flavours, and shake them well before mixing:

TPA Honeydew 3%

TPA Cantaloupe 4%

TPA Kiwi Double 4%

TPA Coconut Extra 0,35%

CAP Italian Lemon Sicily 2%

FA Custard 2%

FA Marshmallow 1%

CAP Super Sweet 0,75%

3. Shake well and place your bottle of e-liquid in a dark place for 14-21 days. Enjoy vaping your new e-juice!

MANDARIN ICE CREAM

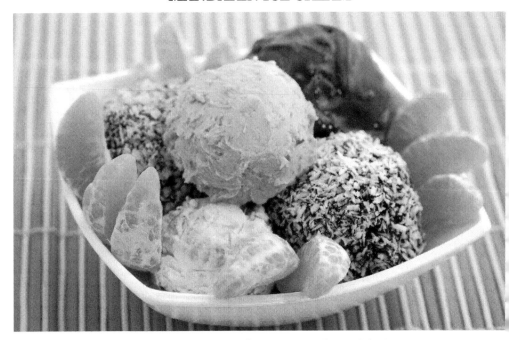

1. Grab your nic base. We recommend you use 70/30 VG/PG.

2. Add these flavours, and shake them well before mixing:

FW Blood Orange 6%

CAP Sweet Tangerine 2%

TPA Coconut Extra 0,35%

FA Vienna Cream 3%

FA Fresh Cream 1,5%

FA Cardamom 0,5%

FA Bergamot 0,5%

FA Marshmallow 1%

CAP Super Sweet 0,75%

3. Shake well and place your bottle of e-liquid in a dark place for 21 days. Enjoy vaping your new e-juice!

CITRUS PUNCH

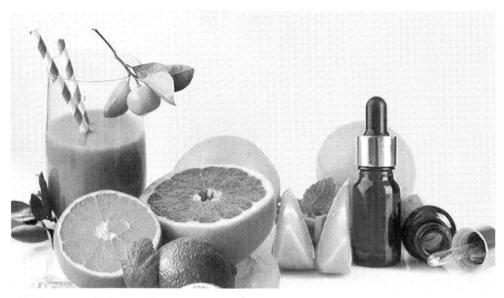

1. Grab your nic base. We recommend you use 70/30 VG/PG.

2. Add these flavours, and shake them well before mixing:

TPA Citrus Punch* 7%

CAP Italian Lemon Sicily 2%

FW Beetle Juice 2%

CAP Lemon Lime 1%

FA Polar Blast 1% or TPA Koolada 1%

* Taste good but needs a long steep.

3. Shake well and place your bottle of e-liquid in a dark place for 21 days. Enjoy vaping your new e-juice!

TROPICAL BEETLES

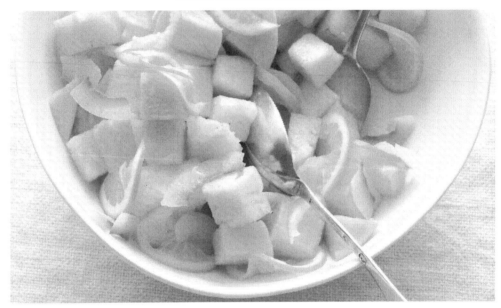

1. Grab your nic base. We recommend you use 70/30 VG/PG.

2. Add these flavours, and shake them well before mixing:

CAP Sweet Mango 5,5%

TPA Dragonfruit 0,75%

CAP Golden Pineapple 2%

FA Custard 1%

FW Beetle Juice 2%

FA Cardamom 0,5%

FA Marshmallow 1%

CAP Super Sweet 0,75%

3. Shake well and place your bottle of e-liquid in a dark place for 21 days. Enjoy vaping your new e-juice!

ALL DAY VAPE! TROPICAL MIX

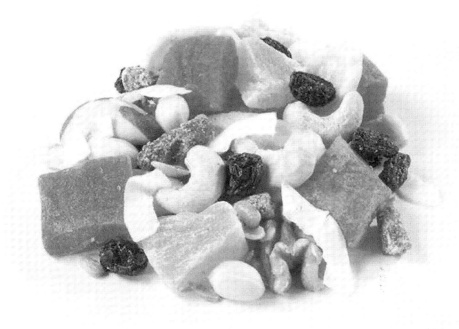

1. Grab your nic base. We recommend you use 70/30 VG/PG.

2. Add these flavours, and shake them well before mixing:

FA Torrone 3%

FA Mandarin 4%

FA Walnut 1%

FA Mango 2%

FA Cardamom 0,5%

TPA Dragonfruit 0,75%

FA Marshmallow 1%

CAP Super Sweet 0,75%

TPA Acetyl Pyrazine 5 PG 1%

3. Shake well and place your bottle of e-liquid in a dark place for 21 days. Enjoy vaping your new e-juice!

FIZZY ORANGE ICE CREAM SODA

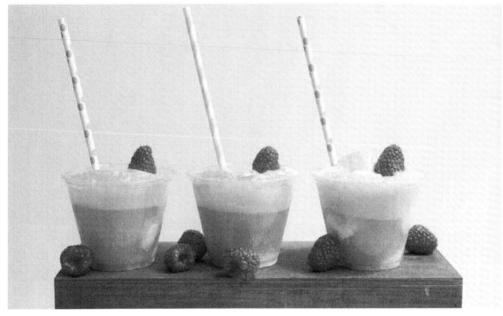

1. Grab your nic base. We recommend you use 70/30 VG/PG.

2. Add these flavours, and shake them well before mixing:

CAP Orange Creamsicle 10%

FA Mandarin 4% or FW Blood Orange 4%

CAP Lemon Lime 1%

TPA Champagne 1%

FA Bergamot 0,5%

TPA Whipped Cream 3%

3. Shake well and place your bottle of e-liquid in a dark place for 21 days. Enjoy vaping your new e-juice!

PINEMANGO CUSTARD

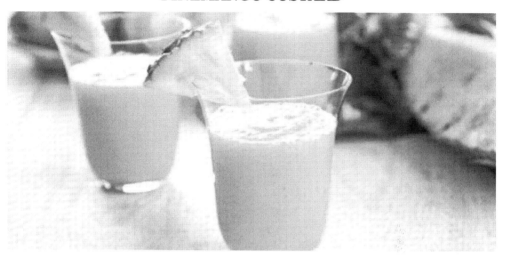

1. Grab your nic base. We recommend you use 70/30 VG/PG.

2. Add these flavours, and shake them well before mixing:

CAP Golden Pineapple 5%

CAP Sweet Mango 5,5%

CAP Coconut 1%

FA Catalan Cream 3%

FA Cream Fresh 1%

FA Vienna Cream 2%

FA Custard 2%

FA Marshmallow 1%

CAP Super Sweet 0,75%

3. Shake well and place your bottle of e-liquid in a dark place for 21 days. Enjoy vaping your new e-juice!

TROPICAL RECIPE FOR BEGINNERS

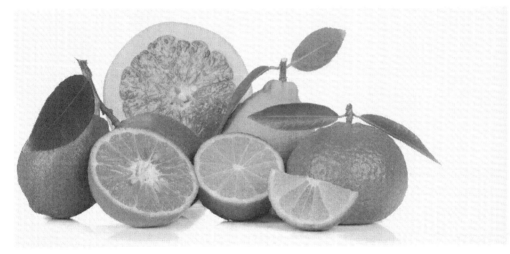

1. Grab your nic base. We recommend you use 70/30 VG/PG.

2. Add these flavours, and shake them well before mixing:

CAP Sweet Guava 6%

TPA Dragonfruit 2%

FA Polar Blast 0,5% or TPA Koolada 0,5%

3. Shake well and place your bottle of e-liquid in a dark place for 21 days. Enjoy vaping your new e-juice

ADVANCED TROPICAL RECIPE

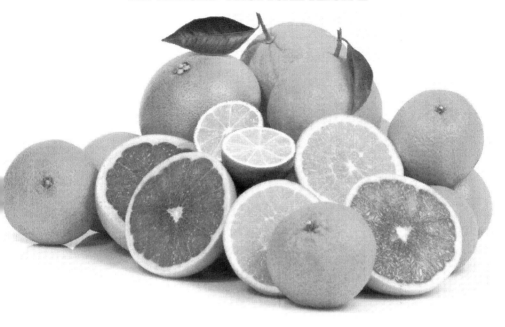

1. Grab your nic base. We recommend you use 70/30 VG/PG.

2. Add these flavours, and shake them well before mixing:

CAP Sweet Tangerine 3%

CAP Sweet Mango 3%

FW Beetle Juice 2%

TPA Dragonfruit 2%

CAP Lemon Lime 1%

FA Lemon Sicily 0,3%

FA Cardamom 0,5%

CAP Super Sweet 0,5%

FA Polar Blast 0,75% or TPA Koolada 0,75%

**3. Shake well and place your bottle of e-liquid in a dark place for 21 days.
Enjoy vaping your new e-juice!**

MR. FRESH FRUIT

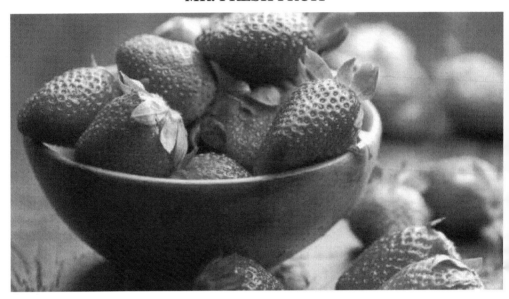

1. Grab your nic base. We recommend you use 70/30 VG/PG.

2. Add these flavours, and shake them well before mixing:

CAP Sweet Guava 6%

CAP Sweet Strawberry 3%

TPA Strawberry Ripe 2%

FA Lemon Sicily 0,3%

TPA Banana Cream 2%

TPA Coconut Extra 0,35%

FA Marshmallow 1%

CAP Super Sweet 0,75%

3. Shake well and place your bottle of e-liquid in a dark place for 21 days. Enjoy vaping your new e-juice!

YO! FRESH ME!

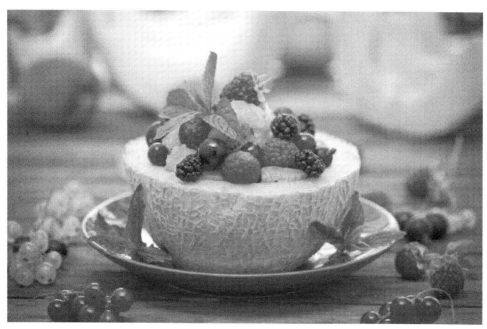

1. Grab your nic base. We recommend you use 70/30 VG/PG.

2. Add these flavours, and shake them well before mixing:

FA Forest Mix 4%

FA Brandy 1%

FA Liquid Amber 0,5%

TPA Honeydew 5%

FA Lemon Sicily 0,5%

TPA Dragonfruit 0,75%

CAP Lemon Lime 1%

FA Polar Blast 0,5% or TPA Koolada 0,5%

3. Shake well and place your bottle of e-liquid in a dark place for 21 days. Enjoy vaping your new e-juice!

PERFECT SUNSET

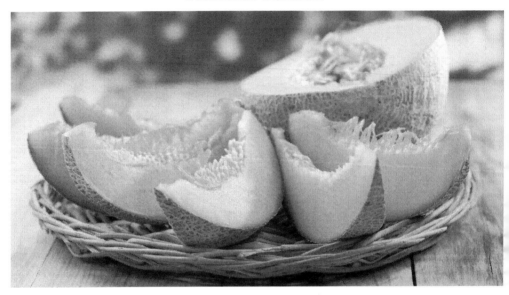

1. Grab your nic base. We recommend you use 70/30 VG/PG.

2. Add these flavours, and shake them well before mixing:

CAP Cantaloupe 5%

CAP Sweet Guava 5%

TPA Banana Cream 6%

FA Lemon Sicily 0,3%

TPA Dragonfruit 0,75%

FA Marshmallow 1%

CAP Super Sweet 0,75%

FA Polar Blast 1% or TPA Koolada 1%

3. Shake well and place your bottle of e-liquid in a dark place for 21 days. Enjoy vaping your new e-juice!

CRANBERRY JAM

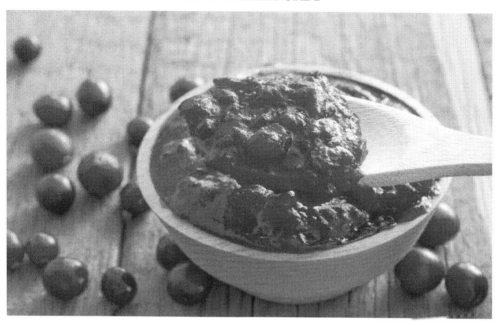

1. Grab your nic base. We recommend you use 70/30 VG/PG.

2. Add these flavours, and shake them well before mixing:

TPA Cranberry Sauce 6%

CAP Raspberry v2 2%

FA Butterscotch 0,5%

TPA Malted Milk 0,5%

FA Custard 2%

FA Marshmallow 1%

CAP Super Sweet 0,75%

3. Shake well and place your bottle of e-liquid in a dark place for 21 days. Enjoy vaping your new e-juice!

FRUITY MADNESS

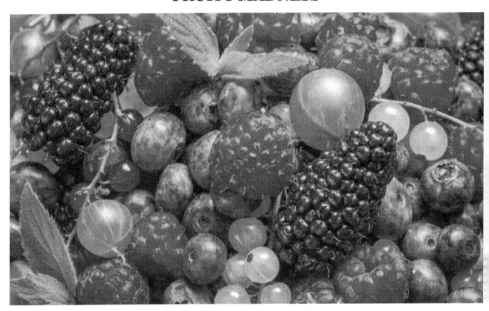

1. Grab your nic base. We recommend you use 70/30 VG/PG.

2. Add these flavours, and shake them well before mixing:

FA Forest Mix 8%

TPA Citrus Punch 6%

FA Lemon Sicily 0,3%

FA Oba Oba 2%

3. Shake well and place your bottle of e-liquid in a dark place for 21 days. Enjoy vaping your new e-juice!

PEACHES YOGURT

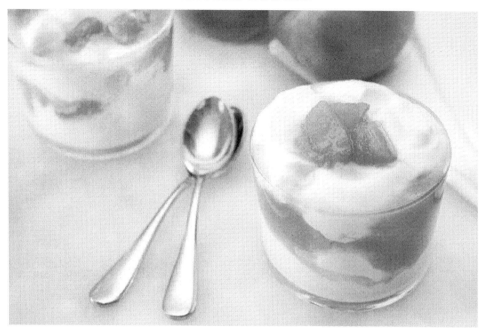

1. Grab your nic base. We recommend you use 70/30 VG/PG.

2. Add these flavours, and shake them well before mixing:

CAP Peaches and Cream 6% or TPA Nectarine 6%

CAP Creamy Yogurt 2%

TPA Whipped Cream 2%

FA Custard 2%

FA Cardamom 0,5%

FA Marshmallow 1%

CAP Super Sweet 0,75%

3. Shake well and place your bottle of e-liquid in a dark place for 21 days. Enjoy vaping your new e-juice!

CHAPTER 6: CANDY FLAVORED E-JUICES

POPCORN

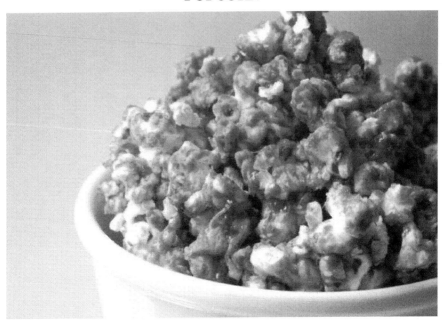

1. Grab your nic base. We recommend you use 70/30 VG/PG.

2. Add these flavours, and shake them well before mixing:

TPA Popcorn 10%

FA Caramel 1% or FW Salted Caramel 3%

FA Cream Fresh 1%

FA Vienna Cream 2%

FA Marshmallow 1%

CAP Super Sweet 0,75%

TPA Acetyl Pyrazine 5 PG 0,5%

3. Shake well and place your bottle of e-liquid in a dark place for 14-21 days. Enjoy vaping your new e-juice!

COLA GUMMY BEARS

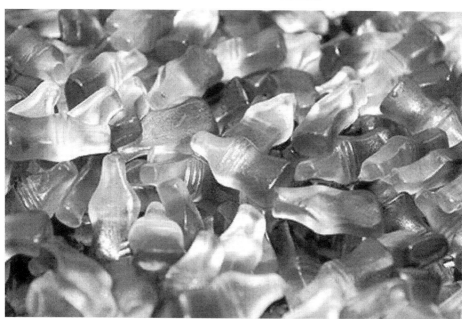

1. Grab your nic base. We recommend you use 70/30 VG/PG.

2. Add these flavours, and shake them well before mixing:

FA Cola 4%

FA Black Cherry 2%

CAP 27 Bears 5%

3. Shake well and place your bottle of e-liquid in a dark place for 21 days. Enjoy vaping your new e-juice!

JUICY GUMMY WORMS

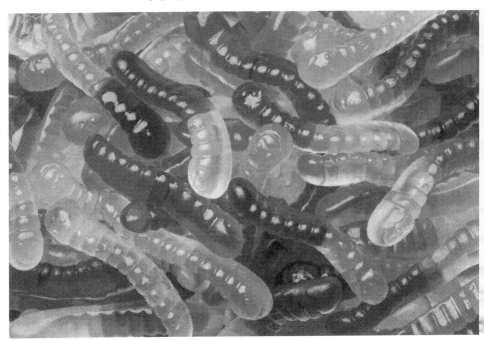

1. Grab your nic base. We recommend you use 70/30 VG/PG.

2. Add these flavours, and shake them well before mixing:

CAP 27 Fish 5% or CAP 27 Bears 5%

CAP Juicy Orange 2%

FA Fuji 2%

FA Lemon Sicily 0,3%

TPA Key Lime 1,5%

FA Sour Wizard 1%

3. Shake well and place your bottle of e-liquid in a dark place for 21 days. Enjoy vaping your new e-juice!

BLUE RASPBERRY GUMMY SMURF

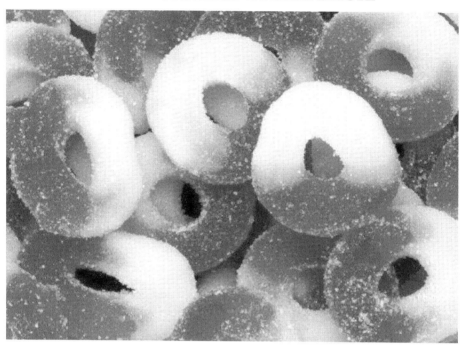

1. Grab your nic base. We recommend you use 70/30 VG/PG.

2. Add these flavours, and shake them well before mixing:

CAP 27 Bears 5% or CAP Jelly Candy 4%

CAP Blue Raspberry Cotton Candy* 7%

TPA Key Lime 1,5%

*As your temperature gets higher, the raspberry notes get increasingly more intense.

3. Shake well and place your bottle of e-liquid in a dark place for 21 days. Enjoy vaping your new e-juice!

SWEDISH FISHES (REMIX)

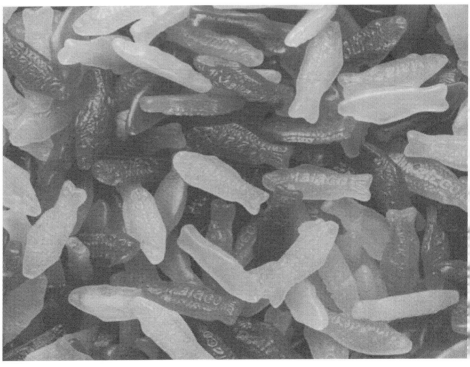

1. Grab your nic base. We recommend you use 70/30 VG/PG.

2. Add these flavours, and shake them well before mixing:

CAP 27 Fish 7%

CAP Jelly Candy 3%

FW Beetle Juice 3%

TPA Key Lime 1,5%

FA Sour Wizard 1%

3. Shake well and place your bottle of e-liquid in a dark place for 21 days. Enjoy vaping your new e-juice!

JELLY PEACHES

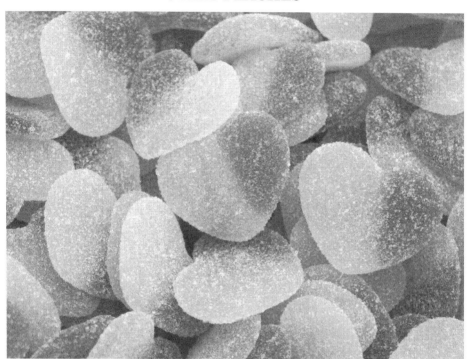

1. Grab your nic base. We recommend you use 70/30 VG/PG.

2. Add these flavours, and shake them well before mixing:

CAP 27 Bears 5%

FA Summer Clouds 1,8%

FA White Peach 2%

TPA Key Lime 1,5%

3. Shake well and place your bottle of e-liquid in a dark place for 21 days. Enjoy vaping your new e-juice!

BLUEBERRY BUBBLEGUM

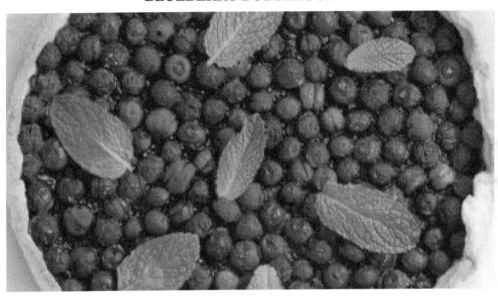

1. Grab your nic base. We recommend you use 70/30 VG/PG.

2. Add these flavours, and shake them well before mixing:

TPA Bubblegum 8%

TPA Blueberry Extra 4%

TPA Blueberry Wild 3%

FA Polar Blast 0,5% or TPA Koolada 0,5%

3. Shake well and place your bottle of e-liquid in a dark place for 21 days. Enjoy vaping your new e-juice!

CIRCUS COTTON CANDY

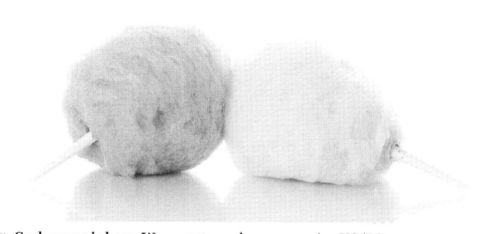

1. Grab your nic base. We recommend you use 70/30 VG/PG.

2. Add these flavours, and shake them well before mixing:

CAP Blue Raspberry Cotton Candy* 8%

TPA Dragonfruit 4%

FA Caramel 1%

*As your temperature gets higher, the raspberry notes get increasingly more intense.

3. Shake well and place your bottle of e-liquid in a dark place for 21 days. Enjoy vaping your new e-juice!

CHAPTER 7: MAMASITA – FITNESS E-JUICE SERIES

MAMASITA: HEALTHY MORNING

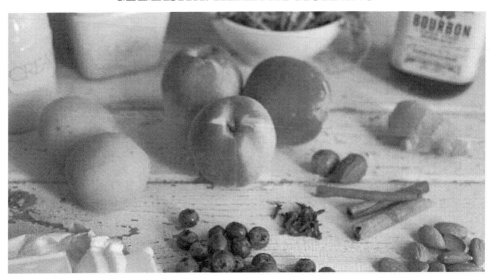

1. Grab your nic base. We recommend you use 70/30 VG/PG.

2. Add these flavours, and shake them well before mixing:

CAP Apricot 4,0%

TPA Apple 6%

FA Nut Mix 2%

FA Catalan Cream 3%

CAP Peaches and Cream 5%

FA Lemon Sicily 0,5%

FA Cinnamon Ceylon 0,5%

FA Maple Syrup 0,25%

TPA Acetyl Pyrazine 5 PG 1%

3. Shake well and place your bottle of e-liquid in a dark place for 21 days. Enjoy vaping your new e-juice!

MAMASITA: LOW-FAT CINNAMON PEACH BANANA BREAD

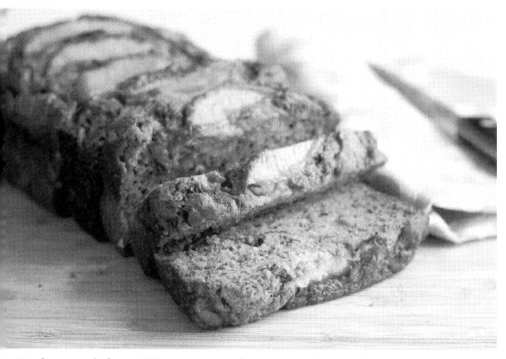

1. Grab your nic base. We recommend you use 70/30 VG/PG.

2. Add these flavours, and shake them well before mixing:

TPA Banana Nut Bread 6%

FA White Peach 0,75%

TPA Peach (Juicy) 3%

FA Liquid Amber 0,5%

FA Catalan Cream 2%

FA Nut Mix 2%

FA Cinnamon Ceylon 0,5%

FA Marshmallow 1%

CAP Super Sweet 0,75%

TPA Acetyl Pyrazine 5 PG 1%

3. Shake well and place your bottle of e-liquid in a dark place for 21 days. Enjoy vaping your new e-juice!

MAMASITA: CINNAMON LOVERS

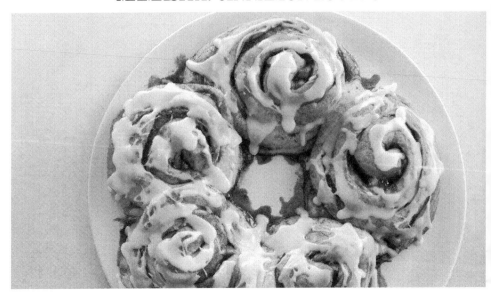

1. Grab your nic base. We recommend you use 70/30 VG/PG.

2. Add these flavours, and shake them well before mixing:

CAP Cinnamon Danish Swirl V2 4%

FA Cookie 1%

FA Apple Pie 4%

CAP Vanilla Custard 4%

FA Marshmallow 1%

CAP Super Sweet 0,75%

TPA Acetyl Pyrazine 5 PG 1%

3. Shake well and place your bottle of e-liquid in a dark place for 21 days. Enjoy vaping your new e-juice!

APRICOT & PECAN VEGAN PANCAKES

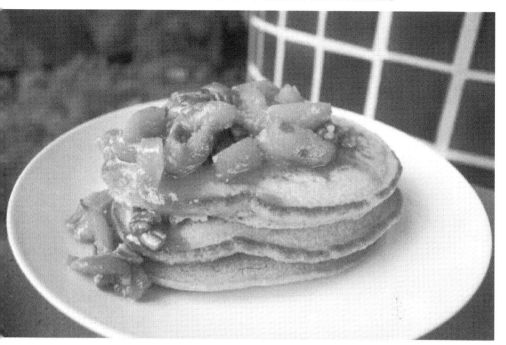

1. Grab your nic base. We recommend you use 70/30 VG/PG.

2. Add these flavours, and shake them well before mixing.

TPA Pancakes 2%

CAP Golden Butter 0,5%

FA Torrone 0,5%

TPA Apricot 2%

CAP Sweet Tangerine 1%

FA Liquid Amber 0,5%

FA Brandy 0,5%

FW Butter Pecan 3%

FA Marshmallow 1%

FA Maple Syrup 0,25%

TPA Acetyl Pyrazine 5 PG 0,75%

3. Shake well and place your bottle of e-liquid in a dark place for 21-28 days. Enjoy vaping your new e-juice!

MAMASITA: CHOCOLATE CHIP COOKIE ICE CREAM SANDWICHES

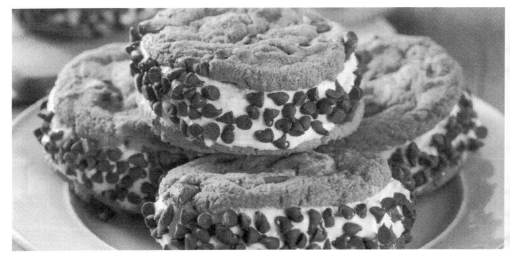

1. Grab your nic base. We recommend you use 70/30 VG/PG.

2. Add these flavours, and shake them well before mixing:

FA Cookie 2%

TPA Cheesecake (Graham Crust) 3%

FW Milk Chocolate 4%

FA Cream Fresh 1%

FA Vienna Cream 2%

FA Custard 2%

FA Marshmallow 1%

CAP Super Sweet 0,75%

TPA Acetyl Pyrazine 5 PG 1%

3. Shake well and place your bottle of e-liquid in a dark place for 28 days. Enjoy vaping your new e-juice!

CHAPTER 8: EXPERIMENTAL RECIPES - YOU EITHER LOVE IT OR HATE IT

FROZEN ROOT BEER [ICE SCREAM]

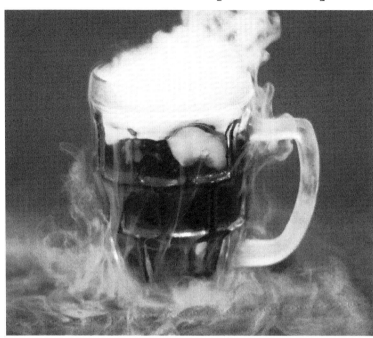

1. Grab your nic base. We recommend you use 70/30 VG/PG.

2. Add these flavours, and shake them well before mixing:

TPA Rootbeer Float 6%

TPA Vanilla Bean Ice Cream 4%

CAP Vanilla Custard v1 0,5%

TPA Champagne 1%

FA Butterscotch 2%

TPA Red Oak 1,5%

FA Oak Wood 0,5%

TPA Koolada 10 PG 1,25%

3. Shake well and place your bottle of e-liquid in a dark place from 25 to 40 days. Enjoy vaping your new e-juice!

PURPLE LAMBORGHINI [MONTH+ STEEP]

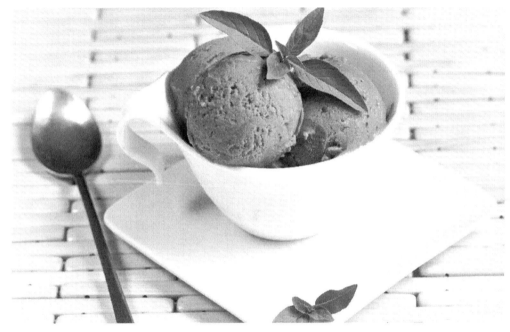

1. Grab your nic base. We recommend you use 70/30 VG/PG.

2. Add these flavours, and shake them well before mixing:

TPA Taro 2%

TPA Coconut Extra 0,25%

TPA Blueberry Extra 4%

TPA Blueberry Wild 3%

FA Cream Fresh 1%

FA Vienna Cream 2%

FA Custard 2%

FA Marshmallow 1%

TPA Koolada 10 PG 0,5%

3. Shake well and place your bottle of e-liquid in a dark from 25 to 40 days. Enjoy vaping your new e-juice!

VAPE THE SLIMER

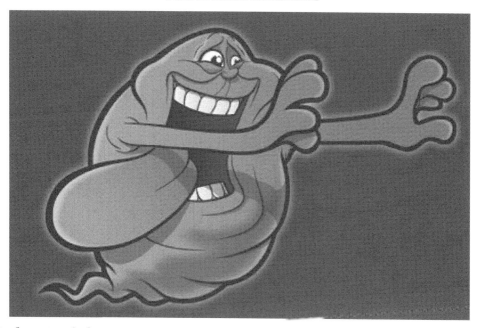

1. Grab your nic base. We recommend you use 70/30 VG/PG.

2. Add these flavours, and shake them well before mixing:

TPA Watermelon 4%

TPA Key Lime 1,5%

CAP Cool Mint 1%

CAP Cucumber 3% or TPA Cucumber 3% or FA Cucumber 0,5%

TPA Cantaloupe 5%

TPA Dragonfruit 0,75%

3. Shake well and place your bottle of e-liquid in a dark place for 21 days. THEN MEET SLIMER!

BONUS! TIRAMISU WITH RASPBERRY JAM

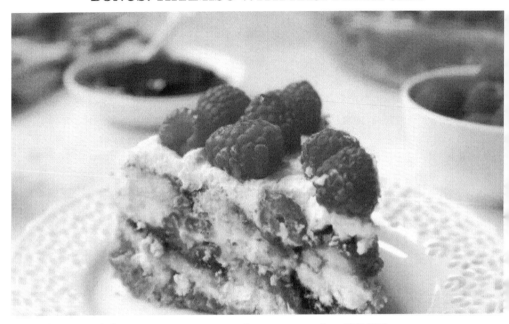

1. Grab your nic base. We recommend you use 70/30 VG/PG.

2. Add these flavours, and shake them well before mixing:

FW Cake Batter Dip 6%

FA Vienna Cream 2%

FA Fresh Cream 1%

FA Tiramisu 2%

FA Lemon Sicily 0,3%

CAP Raspberry v2 1,5%

FA Marshmallow 1%

CAP Super Sweet 0,75%

TPA Acetyl Pyrazine 5 PG 1%

3. Shake well and place your bottle of e-liquid in a dark place for 28 days. Enjoy vaping your new e-juice!

CONCLUSION

Thank you again for purchasing this book, I hope you have enjoyed it!

Could I ask you a favor? If you did enjoy this book, could leave me a review on Amazon? If you search for my name and the title on Amazon you will find it. Thank you so much, it is very much appreciated!

Printed in Great Britain
by Amazon